Recreational Drugs and Drugs Used to Treat Addicted Mothers:

Impact on Pregnancy and Breastfeeding

Frank J. Nice, RPh, DPA, CPHP

Amy C. Luo, RPh, Pharm D

Cheryl A. Harrow, DNP, FNP-BC, IBCLC

Recreational Drugs and Drugs Used to Treat Addicted Mothers: Impact on Pregnancy and Breastfeeding

Frank J. Nice, RPh, DPA, CPHP

Amy C. Luo, RPh, Pharm D

Cheryl A. Harrow, DNP, FNP-BC, IBCLC

© Copyright 2017

Nice Breastfeeding, LLC

7409 Algona Court

Derwood, MD 20855

301-840-0270 phone

301-840-0270 fax

www.NiceBreastfeeding.com

Library of Congress Control Number:

ISBN-13:9780998502403

Table of Contents

Tables and Figures

Tables

Figures

Dedication

This book is dedicated, first of all, to all mothers and fathers who have given birth to or adopted precious children and to all breastfeeding mothers and their children and families. Also, we dedicate this book to all fellow healthcare professionals who dedicate their lives to mothers, fathers, and children.

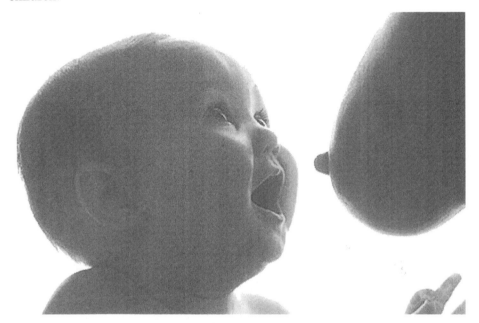

This is now the fourth breastfeeding book that I have authored. I have dedicated my previous books to my Polish ancestors who are the substance of who and what I am now. As some of you know, I have dedicated 40 years of my life to the breastfeeding community, Polish and non-Polish. For the past 20 years, I have also dedicated my professional career to providing medical and pharmaceutical care to the poorest of the poor in Haiti. Having been to Haiti so many times now, I recently was told that I am now a honorary Haitian citizen. Being Polish makes that designation even more significant to me. So once again I dedicate this book to my Polish ancestors, especially to those who lost their lives fighting for the freedom of the Haitian slaves. Here is the rest of the story:

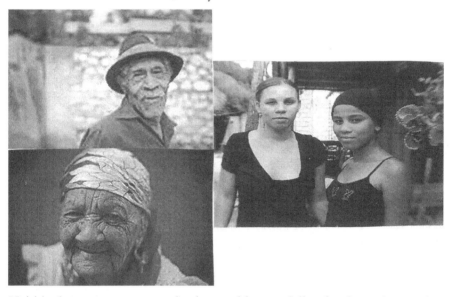

Haiti is the poorest country in the world, especially after its major earthquake in 2010. Haiti, the size of Maryland, is one of the most densely populated countries in the world, with a population of approximately ten million people.

What is extraordinary has been the handful of times I have come face to face with blue-eyed (oh, how those blue eyes shine and reflect back into your heart and soul) Haitian or a Haitian with a Polish sounding name. There is even a village in Haiti called Kasel (Cazale). How did that ever happen?

Haiti was the third country in the world in 1804 to establish a democratic form of government after the world's only successful slave revolution (except for the Jews under Moses). The first democratic government was the United States in 1776, followed by Poland in 1779. How is that for a democratic triumvirate: United States, Poland, and Haiti? During the years to follow, all three nations became intertwined in political intrigue—good and bad.

In 1804, the black slaves of Haiti rose up and went to war against Napoleon and his French Army. When the French forces came to Haiti to suppress the revolution and to fight against the slaves, there were 5,200 Polish Officers and Legionnaires aligned with the French Army.

The Poles were astonished and horrified by the way the Blacks were oppressed, brutalized, ill-equipped, and out-numbered by the French troops. Most of the Polish Legionnaires defected and decided to fight with the Haitian slaves against the Napoleonic forces. Eventually, the Haitian slaves and Polish Legionnaires defeated Napoleon's soldiers, and Haiti became a free and independent democratic nation.

The conflict cost over 4,000 of the Polish Legionnaires their lives. To make matters worse for the Legionnaires, once the French Army lost the war, it returned to France. Many of the surviving Polish Legionnaires were abandoned to stay in Haiti with no way out. They settled in Kasel (Cazale), Jacmel, and Fond des Blancs. They intermarried with Haitian women, and Polish descendants are still there 210 years later. Even though Polish is no longer spoken, there are still those who have Polish names. Maybe, just maybe, you will travel to Haiti and meet one of my fellow Poles.

Frank J. Nice

Growing up, my mother made it seem like breastfeeding was the only way to feed an infant. I do not remember my intimate moments with mom. Luckily, she gave my younger brother the same royal treatment. She was never shy about having me around while she breastfed. I did not appreciate this natural act of breastfeeding as a child. How else would my baby brother eat? Only in pharmacy school, did I learn about mothers giving up breastfeeding soon after birth. Others never intend to breastfeed. Yet, there is another group of mothers I never considered. These are the mothers who want to breastfeed, but healthcare providers advise them not to. Breastfeeding is multifaceted. Mothers have to decide to care for the duo, decide to start breastfeeding, decide to continue, and decide to wean. I would like to dedicate this book to my mother, because she decided to love me.

"This is a breast pump, and it feels different from feeding a baby," said Arija, who has been my best friend since high school. Arija was not shy about demonstrating how she fed her baby. Somehow, she knew a few years in advance that we had to get over this phase. During the 2008 Japan-China trip Arija planned with her now husband, we visited an onsen* (温泉). Basic onsen etiquette dictates entering the bath water without any form of clothing. You thought right. We saw each other naked. The awkward, uncomfortable, laughing-as-a-defense-mechanism feelings did not last long. We relaxed in the hot spring, chatted away, and ended up rejuvenated. Arija got married and gave birth to her daughter a few years later. When I visited her, she was prepared to answer my many questions about breastfeeding. She shared her experience in a patient and gentle way. She understood me when I said babies scare me. She never made me feel guilty when I declined to hold her baby. She helped me become more comfortable with babies, with the way they feed, with the idea of being a mother. In fact, I voluntarily asked to hold her second baby when I visited her recently! I would like to dedicate this book to Arija. Because of you, I can now relate to my patients better.

When Dr. Nice (he tells me to call him Frank, but I continue to call him 'doctor' behind his back) approached me to write this book, I was ecstatic: a book deal! Dr. Nice is an expert in the field of medications and breastfeeding. His confidence in me to work alongside him took me by surprise. I am grateful that he chooses to share his years of experience and knowledge with me. He continues to serve as my mentor: encouraging me, supporting me, inspiring me. Thus, I would like to dedicate this book to him.

*In case you were wondering, the onsen ryokan had single sex pools.

Amy C. Luo

Acknowledgements

The older I get, the more I am encouraged and driven by the family God has given and continues to give me here on earth. Without the gift and presence of family, there would be no drive to accomplish things like writing books, among many others. Having said that, I simply acknowledge:

Grandparents: Philip and Sophia Nice; George and Katherine Kuscavage

Parents: Frank, Sr., and Irene

Siblings: Lillian, Bill, and Kathy

Wife: Myung Hee

Children: Franus', Melania, Eryk, Liana, Sue, and Bryan

Grandchildren: Aaron, Abigail, Acadia, Amaris, Benjamin, Caitlin, Elijah, and Evan

God has truly blessed me.

Frank J. Nice

To my mother Feifen: Without you breastfeeding me, I'd be less than I am today.

To my best friend Arija: Without going to a Japanese *onsen* (hot spring) with you, watching you breastfeed your little ones would still be an awkward experience.

(Kendall, that means we got over that awkward turtle, too.)

Amy C. Luo

Special Thanks

The authors are most grateful for the extremely important and extensive contribution of **Cheryl A. Harrow**, DNP, FNP-BC, IBCLC, for guest authoring Chapter 8: Neonatal Abstinence Syndrome (NAS).

Dr. Cheryl Ann Harrow has practiced as a nurse, nurse practitioner, educator, consultant, lecturer, and author on neonatal abstinence syndrome and breastfeeding over the past 40 years. She holds a Bachelor of Science in Nursing Degree, a Master of Science Degree, and a Doctorate in Nursing Practice. Dr. Harrow has been a Family Nurse Practitioner for over 15 years, an International Board Certified Lactation Consultant for over 25 years, and holds certification in Low Risk Neonatal Nursing. She is currently a Nurse Practitioner in the Nursery at Johns Hopkins Bayview Medical Center and teaches at The Catholic University of America.

Dr. Harrow is known internationally for her expertise in NAS and lactation. She has participated in numerous research studies and co-authored multiple publications on NAS, as well as both NAS and breastfeeding. She actively participates in the promotion of the pursuit of breastfeeding by opioid-dependent women engaged in counseling and maintenance therapy.

The authors are also deeply appreciative to have the Foreword written by **Philip O. Anderson**, Pharm.D, FASHP, FCSHP. Dr. Anderson is a pharmacist pioneer in the field of medications and breastfeeding. He was one of the first to publish complete findings on medication use during breastfeeding. His defining accomplishment was to author the National Library of Medicine's LactMed database (http://toxnet.nlm.nih.gov/cgi-bin/sis/htmlgen?LACT), which provides information on the use of medications in nursing mothers. Frank J. Nice, the primary author, has had the honor and privilege to know and work with Dr. Anderson over the many years of our careers.

The authors also wish to give special thanks to the following colleagues for helping to provide vignettes for inclusion in our book:

Laurie Beck, IBCLC, RLC

Katherine Brown, SBD, CLD, CCE, CBS

Betty Crase, LLLI

Alison Grady, IBCLC, RLC

Angela Kirkwood, RN, BSN, IBCLC, RLC

Nikki Lee, MS, IBCLC, CCE, CIMI, ANLC, CKC

James J. McKenna, PhD

Sheila J. Norman

Jeanette Panchula, BSW, RN, PHN, IBCLC

Linda Pohl, IBCLC, RLC

Tonse N. K. Raju, MD, DCH

Julie Tardos, IBCLC

Tonya Hardney Vela

The authors especially wish to give special thanks to **"Brianna,"** a very special mother. From the depths of her heart, Brianna revealed what resides in the heart of a mother who becomes pregnant while using recreational drugs and then fights the battle for what is best for her breastfed baby and for any future pregnancies.

Foreword

A new drug is created. It goes through animal testing, then, if safe, it goes through testing in humans to find the proper dosage and to see how it should be used and not used. This information is critically evaluated and summarized in a package insert distributed with the drug. Wouldn't it be great if drugs of abuse went through this process? Unfortunately, they do not. What we have instead are bits and pieces of information, often based on adverse effects or outright disasters that occurred with uncontrolled use of these substances.

The healthcare provider is thrust into this minefield of unknowns when encountering a pregnant or breastfeeding patient who is using a substance of abuse. Some clinicians may refuse to deal with these women, while others rely on limited personal experience or snippets of information picked up from others during their careers.

Frank Nice and his colleagues have addressed this lack of information for those who deal with pregnant and nursing mothers with substance abuse issues. This book brings the medication expertise of pharmacists together with the expertise of experienced clinicians of other disciplines. It sets down guidelines from professional organizations into one place to rationally assess the information that is available, while putting them into an organized and useable context. Case vignettes sprinkled throughout the chapters provide a sense of the "real world" that the reader may encounter in practice.

No book of this nature can ever be entirely complete or cover every possible situation because of the uncontrolled nature of substance abuse and lack of high-quality information. Nevertheless, the authors have done well in creating a rational framework that can guide clinical decision-making. This book should serve well as a starting point for inexperienced clinicians and a solid resource for more experienced practitioners who may not have the formal pharmacologic background that the authors bring to the discussion.

Philip O. Anderson, Pharm.D., FASHP, FCSHP

Health Sciences Clinical Professor of Pharmacy

University of California San Diego

Skaggs School of Pharmacy and Pharmaceuticals Sciences

Introduction

Frank J. Nice

Brianna's Story - Background

Brianna (not her real name), is a 36-year-old female (at the time of the birth), with an unplanned pregnancy with her new boyfriend (who was also addicted to narcotic painkillers). She had a yoga injury at a time in her life when she would not take Advil for pain, so she did not go to the doctor for five years.

By the time she saw a physician, she was in severe pain and almost unable to work. She was addicted to Dilaudid and other narcotics after a neck/back injury over six years ago. She had surgery the year before conception that used part of her hip bone to fuse her cervical spine. She was told there would be a two-year recovery. She accidentally got pregnant a year after the surgery. At the time of conception, she had probably been on narcotics on-and-off for over two years, with a gradually increasing dose. She was unable to wean off the medication or stop during early pregnancy. When her prescription ran out, she bought OxyContin, Percocet, or other narcotics off the street, as she could, until she could refill again. She was discharged from her current pain management clinic because it did not see pregnant women. She was transferred to a different clinic that worked with her hospital and OB, yet one with not as good a reputation.

(Name withheld by request; used with permission)

(Continued in Chapter 1)

Looking Back

Since the creation of our first parents, human life has been sustained by pregnancies and breastfeeding, especially breastfeeding. There was no artificial formula to sustain mankind throughout most of its history. As the history of mankind progressed, the use and ingestion of recreational substances, natural drug substances, and synthetic drugs and their abuse followed. There is no history of when the first pregnant woman or first breastfeeding woman used recreational substances, unknowingly ingested a potentially harmful food or herbal, or knowingly used a drug of abuse. It is quite apparent that in our current society, pregnant and breastfeeding women do use and ingest recreational substances (in both a wise and unwise manner) and drugs of abuse, natural and/or synthetic. Because they do, there is also a direct need to treat those mothers and their babies who become addicted. As we progress with this book, the stories and the statistics will stand out.

We need not be defined by the past use of medications and drugs, including recreational and drugs of abuse, during pregnancy and breastfeeding, but we can certainly be prepared and learn from their past use. It is the authors' goal to present the current knowledge, understanding, and wisdom on the use of recreational drugs and drugs of abuse, and the drug methods used to treat addicted mothers and their impact on pregnancy and breastfeeding. As the primary author, I have 40 years of intimate experience working with the breastfeeding community. My experience with pregnancy has been more limited and mainly a related outgrowth of my breastfeeding experiences. I have developed many medication and breastfeeding methodologies, counseling tools and techniques, and algorithms for drug use during breastfeeding, and authored several books and over 50 journal articles. Thus, the contents of this book will, by necessity, be weighted to the breastfeeding side of the equation. Despite this, medication use during pregnancy will be given its due. In fact, many times we will compare and contrast the use of medications in pregnancy with their use in breastfeeding. Hopefully, most mothers will breastfeed much longer than they were ever pregnant for both their benefit and their child's benefit.

Chapter 1: An Overview of Medications and Pregnancy: Current Concepts

Frank J. Nice

Brianna's Story - Pregnancy

Brianna took a pregnancy test on a Saturday, and on Monday went to see her primary care doctor. She had been seen for pain management for a year (before and after surgery). She called a homebirth midwife, made an appointment with her, and was told she could not have a homebirth unless she was weaned off drugs completely. *"I wanted to [wean completely]…but at that point I was not able to do it."* Her current pain management doctor would not treat pregnant women. She had trouble finding a doctor who would work with her in terms of weaning completely versus a maintenance dose of narcotics. She switched to an OB office that worked with pain management, attempted to wean, but the schedule was too drastic for her. She was experiencing severe withdrawal symptoms and having to supplement with street drugs.

Brianna felt the maintenance dose prescribed by her OB was way too low, and this caused withdrawal symptoms. She felt her OB then accused her of drug-seeking behavior because she was in withdrawal. *"I was on a bunch of medications, that I stopped that Saturday that I found out [except the Dilaudid]…I feel that the Oxycodone is better for pain relief, but I felt that I never slept on the Oxycodone, so I asked to be switched back to the Dilaudid."*

"I think he [the OB] was profiling me as drug seeking behavior…" Brianna expressed trying to reconcile with herself the fact that the medication worked for pain, but she recognized that she was addicted and did not want to be. Notably, Brianna was not offered any type of addiction counseling while pregnant.

Brianna felt strongly that the maintenance dose given to her during her pregnancy was completely inadequate. They lowered her dose every three days, resulting in withdrawal symptoms during pregnancy. During those times, she would buy narcotics off the street to ease the withdrawal symptoms until her doctors agreed to a maintenance dose that she felt was acceptable.

Brianna's labor was very quick. She was 10 cm and pushing by the time they arrived at the hospital. Baby was born without any interventions. During that time they pulled up her file and she informed them of her narcotic prescription and current intake. She was told that no withdrawal symptoms would present for the first 24 hours.

(Continued in Chapter 2)

Statistics and More Statistics

According to the United States pregnancy statistics for 2014 (1), there were six million pregnancies resulting in the birth of 4,058,000 children. There were issues with 1,955,840 of these pregnancies. Of these, there were 600,000 miscarriages, 64,000 ectopic pregnancies, 6,000 molar pregnancies, and 26,000 stillbirths. Of all pregnancies, 14.5% of women experienced one or more pregnancy complications, 7.7% of children were born prematurely, 5.1% of children had a low birth rate, 2% of babies were born with birth defects, and 0.45% of infants died before their first birthday.

Let us look at some pregnancy statistics related to drug use (2). Data from 1976-2008 (which should closely reflect ongoing data) reported that approximately 90% of women take at least one prescription medication. A 2005 Over-The-Counter (OTC) medications study (which again should closely reflect current use) reported that most women take OTC products. Data from 1998-2004 reported that 10.9% of pregnant women use herbal products. One can reasonably conclude that almost every pregnant woman takes some kind of medication during her pregnancy. Over the past 30 years, prescription drug use in pregnant women has increased more than 60%. First trimester use of four or more medications has nearly tripled, while use of four or more medications anytime during pregnancy has more than doubled.

Here are even more statistics on recreational and illicit drug use (3). During 2012-2013, 5.4% of pregnant women aged 15 to 44 were illicit drug users compared to 11.4% of non-pregnant women. Use was higher during the third trimester than during the first and second trimesters. The highest use of illicit drugs was among women aged 15 to 17, at 14.6%, and lowest for women aged 26 to 44, at 3.2%. Among pregnant women, 8.5% reported alcohol use, 2.7% reported binge drinking, and 0.3% reported heavy drinking compared to 55.5% alcohol use among non-pregnant women. Approximately one in six (15.9%) pregnant women compared to 24.6% of non-pregnant women smoked tobacco. The highest rate of smoking was among pregnant women aged 18-25. While the percentage of women smoking overall has decreased over the past years, the rate among pregnant women has not changed significantly.

These statistics are quite stunning. The affects of recreational and illicit drugs by pregnant women are even more stunning. According to the Academy of Breastfeeding Medicine (ABM) Clinical Protocol #21: Guidelines for Breastfeeding and Substance Use or Substance Use Disorder, revised 2015, illicit drug use and legal substance use/abuse remains a significant problem after the pregnancy when women then breastfeed (4). Illicit drug use presents significant challenges and risks not only for the pregnant woman, but also for the breastfeeding woman. Substance abuse disorders facilitate behaviors and conditions that affect both mother and baby, at birth, soon after birth, and long after birth (5). Such issues as Neonatal Abstinence Syndrome, treatment for opioid dependence, legal ramifications, social concerns, and loss of the benefits of breastfeeding will be covered in later chapters. Specific drug concerns and effects will also be covered.

Multiple drug use and /or abuse are common. In addition to the drugs themselves, dangerous and often unknown adulterants are present in the dosage form or more potent and powerful forms are now available than in the past. Drug users and abusers are at a higher risk for infections, as well as have a higher prevalence for psychiatric disorders, which can lead to further drug overload and cognitive impairment. Making rational healthcare decisions, such as breast is best for her infant, are often difficult and unobtainable. These issues will be discussed further when breastfeeding is more specifically addressed.

Basic Pregnancy Terminology and Characteristics

When discussing drug use during pregnancy, it helps to know basic pregnancy and drug terminology so we all remain on the same level of understanding (6).

Gravidity: The number of pregnancies for a woman regardless of the outcome (multiple births equal single pregnancy)

Parity: Number of deliveries after 20 weeks gestation

> First number is the number of deliveries (37-42 weeks)

> Second number is the number of premature deliveries (before 37 weeks)

> Third number is the number of ectopic or aborted pregnancies

> Fourth number is the number of living children

> **TPAL** is the total Terms, Prematures, Abortions, and Living

Gestation: Period of fetal development in the uterus from conception until birth

Term Delivery:

> **Early Term:** Between 37 weeks 0 days and 38 weeks 6 days

> **Full Term:** Between 39 weeks 0 days and 40 weeks 6 days

> **Late Term:** Between 41 weeks 0 days and 41 weeks 6 days

> **Post Term:** Between 42 weeks and beyond

Term Pregnancy: 37-42 weeks; average is 40 weeks; before 37 weeks is premature; fetus is considered viable at 22-24 weeks

Trimesters:

> **First:** date of Last Menstrual Period (LMP) to week 13

> **Second:** 14-26 weeks

> **Third:** 27 weeks to birth (perinatal)

Due Date: First day of last menses plus one week minus three months

The following are common characteristics of pregnancy:

Amenorrhea (spotting possible)

Nausea and vomiting ("morning" sickness): 2-16 weeks or longer

Frequent urination: 6-8 weeks

Darkening of areola: first trimester

Blue discoloration of vaginal mucosa

Enlarging of uterus and abdomen: 8-12 weeks

Fetal movements: 18-22 weeks

Weight Gain:

> Normal weight pre-pregnancy: 25-35 pounds

> Underweight pre-pregnancy: Up to 40 pounds

> Overweight pre-pregnancy: 15 pounds

Basic Drug Considerations During Pregnancy

Many physiologic and pharmacokinetic changes occur with drug use during pregnancy that affects the pharmacologic actions of the drug. These changes start in the first trimester and peak in the second trimester. Among the most important are:

- Plasma volume, cardiac output, and Glomerular Filtration Rate (GFR) increase 30-50%, which result in decreased concentrations of renally (kidney) eliminated drugs.
- Body fat increases, which increases the Volume of Distribution (Vd) of fat-soluble drugs.
- Albumin decreases, which increases the Vd of protein-bound drugs (unbound drugs are thus metabolized more by the liver and kidneys).
- Altered gastrointestinal (GI) absorption leads to nausea and vomiting, delayed gastric emptying, increased gastric pH, which increases drug concentrations.
- Estrogen and progesterone levels increase, which causes increased hepatic (liver) metabolism of drugs.
- Drugs transfer from mother to child transplacentally (though the placenta).
- Most drugs transfuse between maternal and fetal blood.
- Drugs with a molecular weight/mass of greater than 600 Daltons readily cross the placenta; 600-1,000 Daltons cross more slowly; greater than 1,000 Daltons cross insignificantly.
- Lipophilic (fat soluble) drugs cross more readily than hydrophilic (water soluble) drugs.
- Fetal albumin levels are higher than maternal albumin levels, which result in higher fetal concentrations of highly protein-bound drugs.
- Fetal blood pH is less than maternal pH, which causes weak base drugs to more easily cross the placenta, ionize, and be less likely to diffuse back.
- Only unbound drugs can cross the placenta.
- The placenta is capable of drug metabolism (also true for mammary epithelium).
- Blood flow to the uterus greatly impacts drug transfer to the fetus.

Drug Transfer

Most evidence for evaluating drug use during pregnancy comes from the following sources:

- Animal studies (these studies may be quite difficult to extrapolate to humans)
- Case reports (observational one time or one patient reports)
- Case-controlled studies (retrospective observational studies)
- Cohort studies (observational studies of groups of people with defined characteristics who are followed up to determine incidence

of, or mortality from, some specific disease, all causes of death, or some other outcome)

- Voluntary reporting/registries (note: there are no breastfeeding registries)

When these reports, studies, and registries are evaluated, we need to consider the sample size, maternal disease contribution, recall bias, and confounding variables.

Guidelines

Whenever anyone needs to take medication during pregnancy, just as with breastfeeding, the benefits of the drug must be weighed against the risks of the drug for both the mother and child. No current approved drug produces abnormalities in all exposed fetuses. Teratogenicity is the capability of a drug to produce congenital abnormalities. The overall risk for congenital abnormalities in the general population is approximately 3%. Less than 1% is due to drugs, 15-25% is due to genetics, 10% is environmental, and 65-75% is unknown (which could include drugs). Teratogenicity is impacted by genetic predisposition/genotypes, stage at the time of drug exposure (i.e., trimester), dose of the drug, specificity of the drug, and other simultaneous exposures (which makes drug causation difficult to determine). Teratogenic complications can include: premature/delayed labor, spontaneous abortion, malformations, altered fetal growth, functional deficits, carcinogenesis, and mutagenesis. Neural tube defects, cleft palate/lip, and cardiac abnormalities are the most common major effects.

Guidelines for medication use in pregnancy, as with breastfeeding, include eliminating all nonessential drugs (most crucial); identifying patterns of drug use before conception, if possible; discouraging self-medication, minimizing exposure to harmful drugs (e.g., recreational and illicit); and adjusting doses and dosage forms of medications. Pre-pregnancy treatment considerations can be implemented to help prevent teratogenicity:

- Prenatal vitamins, including 30-65 mg of iron daily to support maternal and fetal erythropoiesis (red cell production). Gastrointestinal upset can worsen nausea and vomiting in the first trimester, but this should not be a reason to discontinue prenatal vitamins treatment.
- Calcium: 1,000-2,000 mg per day to support fetal bone development and prevention of maternal hypertension.
- Folic Acid: to prevent neural tube defects. Treatment should start one month prior to conception and continue through the first trimester. At least 0.4 mg per day should be given pre-pregnancy and

1 mg per day during the pregnancy. Mothers with a history of children with neural tube defects or taking anticonvulsants (especially carbamazepine and valproic acid) should take 4 mg daily.

- Rubella, Hepatitis B, and Influenza prophylaxis

There are many conditions that can occur during pregnancy where the benefits and appropriateness of drug treatment are beneficial for the mother and child. Among these conditions are nausea and vomiting, constipation, gastroesophageal reflux disease (GERD), hemorrhoids, diarrhea, coughs and colds, allergies and allergic rhinitis, essential and gestational hypertension, preeclampsia, eclampsia, gestational diabetes mellitus, coagulation disorders, urinary tract infections, sexually transmitted infections, asthma, epilepsy, human immunodeficiency virus, mental health issues, thyroid issues, preterm labor and tocolysis, labor and delivery complications, labor induction, postpartum hemorrhage, and analgesia. The intent of this book is not to cover the pharmacology and use of these medications during pregnancy. That would be a textbook in itself.

As a practicing pharmacist who knows well that the use of analgesics can be abused and misused, the proper use of analgesics during pregnancy is worth discussing at this point. For the treatment of acute pain, the drug of choice is acetaminophen. Acetaminophen is safe and not teratogenic at normal doses of no more than 3 grams per day, although most patients, pregnant or not, probably should limit daily doses to 2.4 grams per day to avoid any potential toxicity. Opioids and opioids combined with acetaminophen (make sure the patient is not taking any other acetaminophen at the same time) are acceptable at appropriate doses short term. Opioids with prolonged use and/or at high doses are associated with Neonatal Abstinence Syndrome (NAS), which will be discussed in Chapter 8. Non-steroidal Anti-inflammatory Drugs (NSAIDs) at appropriate doses are acceptable for use in the first and second trimesters, but are contraindicated in the third trimester due to their inhibition of labor, negative effect on platelet function, and constriction of the ductus arteriosus.

Pharmacologic analgesia during labor consists of parenteral opioids, epidural blocks (opioid plus or minus an anesthetic, usually Fentanyl plus or minus bupivacaine, and epidurals as Patient Controlled Analgesia (PCA). These agents can prolong the first and second stages of labor and cause headache, often severe, if the subarachnoid space is punctured. Epidural analgesia has a better profile than parenteral opioids, which can result in poorer maternal pain relief and less vigorous neonates. Both can have negative effects on breastfeeding, mainly affecting proper latching by the baby to the breast.

The best analgesia, if possible and worth a try, is the use of nonpharmacologic treatments. These include:

- Warm baths
- Intradermal injections of warm sterile water
- Acupuncture
- Audioanalgesia
- Relaxation
- Breathing techniques
- Heat/cold applications
- Aromatherapy
- Acupressure
- Hypnosis

Summary

The intent of this chapter is to give the reader a general overview on the use of all medications during pregnancy. By understanding the information presented, the reader will have a foundation of information to better understand, evaluate, make recommendations, and counsel pregnant women who are using, misusing, or abusing recreational drugs, "legal" and illegal drug substances, and illicit medications or substances. This will also be true for counseling those mothers who wish to breastfeed their infants after birth.

Chapter 2: An Overview of Medications and Breastfeeding: Current Concepts

Amy C. Luo

Brianna's Story - Breastfeeding

After birth, her baby breastfed very well, was allowed to room in with them initially, and nursed on demand. She nursed exclusively for six months and then started to introduce foods. Her child basically weaned himself by 20 months. By that point, he was basically only nursing at night. (Brianna continued to take narcotic pain medication this entire time, which her doctors told her was okay).

"I was willing to do it on demand too [breastfeeding]."

"I KNOW that the reason that he did not have to take the morphine in the hospital is because of the breastfeeding. And half of it is because of comfort [and the rest from the small amount of drugs that get into the milk]. So he was able to go through almost cold turkey withdrawal at hours, days old, because of nursing."

"Breastfeeding saved my child from having to be in the hospital for a couple weeks. It saved him from a multitude of…aside from all of the regular benefits of breastfeeding and the comfort it offers…"

Brianna was committed to breastfeeding her baby after birth, citing both the comfort and nutrition as her reason for doing so. *"To have to go through withdrawal on top of it [birth], something that I can't do as an adult…"*

(Continued in Chapter 8)

Introduction

In the Jan/Feb 2012 issue of *The Journal of the American Pharmacists Association* (JAPhA), the authors published the seminal article, "Medications and breastfeeding: Current concepts." (1) The main objective of the authors to write the article was to help make this decision by mothers and their healthcare providers a well-educated one, based on objective data and information. The same could be said about the use of illicit and recreational drug substances. An estimated one million mothers every year in the United States decide not to breastfeed, or to discontinue breastfeeding, because of the need to take medication. The article became the most-read article by pharmacists on the topic of breastfeeding and medications, and continues to rank in the Top Ten. As part of an informed discussion on drug use and breastfeeding, the following areas of interest were discussed:

- Pharmacokinetics factors
- Maternal and child factors
- Counseling and the Stepwise Approach
- **Recreational drug use**
- Galactogogues
- OTC medications
- Herbal remedies

Recreational Drug Use

Breast milk retains its quality and composition when the mother (1):

- Has a cold
- Eats junk food
- Suffers malnutrition
- Has a sedentary lifestyle (2)

However, the composition of breast milk is altered when the mother takes drugs that are likely to cross the blood-brain barrier

Recreational drugs are more likely to cross the blood-brain barrier, and are also more likely to cross into breast milk. Crossing the blood-brain barrier is why they are more likely to be abused in the first place. Several reviews and small studies suggest that the immunological, physiological, nutritional, and psychological benefits of breastfeeding outweigh the risk from even natural contaminants. (3, 4, 5, 6) On the other hand, the risk of breastfeeding while using drugs that cross the blood-brain barrier is more complicated and dangerous. (7)

Concentration of Drugs in Breast Milk

The most important pharmacokinetic factors that affect drug substances concentration in breast milk are (1):

- Volume of Distribution (V_d)
    - How widely the substance is distributed in the body.
    - Substances with a high V_d may have lower concentration in the breast milk.

- If the V_d = 1 to 20 L/kg, the substance is likely to pass into milk poorly.

- Percentage (of maternal) Protein Binding (PB)

  o How extensively the substance is bound to the plasma albumin and other proteins.

  o If the **PB > 90%**, the substance is likely to pass into milk poorly.

- Molecular Weight (aka, Molecular Mass) (MW)

  o How likely a substance will pass through mammary epithelium and enter human milk.

  o Substances with higher MWs must be actively transported or dissolved in the cells' lipid membranes.

  o If **MW > 800 Da**, the substance is likely to pass into milk poorly.

These factors are true for legal, recreational, and illicit substances. The following pharmacokinetic factors should also be considered:

- Acidity Measurement (pH)

  o Breast milk is more acidic than plasma.

  o Substances with low pH may have lower concentrations in breast milk than in plasma.

- Partition Coefficient (logP)

  o Breast milk has a higher fat concentration than plasma.

  o Substances with low logP (more water soluble) may have lower concentration in breast milk than in plasma.

- Time of Maximum Concentration (T_{max})

  o Timing breastfeeding sessions to avoid T_{max} of substances can decrease infant exposure.

- Half Life ($t_{1/2}$)

  o Substances with shorter $t_{1/2}$ can decrease infant exposure.

- Milk-to-Plasma Ratio (MP)

  o Ratio of substance concentration in the milk vs. plasma.

  o If **MP < 1**, the substance is likely to pass into milk poorly.

- Active Transport
  - Substances can enter the breast milk via carrier-mediated active transport.
- Relative Infant Dose (RID)
  - Theoretical infant weight-adjusted dose maternal ÷ weight-adjusted dose = good estimate of maternal dose received by the infant.
  - If **RID < 10% of maternal dose**, the substance is likely to pass into milk poorly.

Pharmacokinetic Summary

It is not necessary for the reader to know all the technical terminology of pharmacokinetics used above or in the table below, but any breastfeeding healthcare professional should be able to describe the general concepts when counseling women and interested parties on the use of drugs while breastfeeding. Thus, one can describe the process of the drug molecule being too large to pass into breast milk, or being held or bound more tightly in plasma (blood) than in breast milk, or being too diluted or widely distributed in the mother's body to have much of the drug concentrated in breast milk. On the other hand, the technical terminology is presented if needed by others, such as pharmacists, physicians, researchers, who desire to have theoretical discussions on the use of medications during breastfeeding.

As demonstrated by the Table 2.1 below, recreational drugs vary in pharmacokinetic properties.

Table 2.1 The Pharmacokinetic Properties of Recreational Drugs (8, 9)

Substance	MW (Da)	LogP	V_d (L/Kg)	pK_a*
3,4-methylenedioxymeth-amphetamine/ MDMA (Ecstasy)	193.2423 g/mol	2.28	-	-
3,4-methylenedioxypyro-valeron/MDPV (Bath Salts)	275.34284 g/mol	3.97	-	-

Alprazolam	308.76492 g/mol	2.12	-	40 mg/L at pH 7; 12 mg/mL at pH 1.2
Amphetamine	135.20622 g/mol	1.76	Protein binding and volume of distribution varies widely	10.1 Aqueous solutions are alkaline to litmus.
Benzphetamine	275.81628 g/mol	-	-	-
Buprenorphine	467.64014 g/mol	4.98	188 - 335 L	8.31
Butalbital	224.25634 g/mol	1.87	-	-
Butorphanol	327.46046 g/mol	3.3	305 to 901 L	-
Caffeine	194.1906 g/mol	-0.07	0.8 to 0.9 L/kg [infants]; 0.6 L/kg [adults]	10.4
Camphor	152.23344 g/mol	2.38	Large volume of distribution	-
Carisoprodol	260.32996 g/mol	2.36	-	-

Chloral Hydrate	165.40302 g/mol	0.99	0.6 L/kg	-
Chlordiazepoxide	299.75486 g/mol	2.44	-	4.8
Cocaine	303.35294 g/mol	2.30	Between 1 and 3 L/kg	8.61 Aqueous solutions are alkaline to litmus.
Cocaine (Topical)	303.35294 g/mol	2.30	Between 1 and 3 L/kg	8.61 Aqueous solutions are alkaline to litmus.
Codeine	299.36424 g/mol	1.14	3-6 L/kg	8.21
Cyclobenzaprine**	275.38744 g/mol	5.2	-	8.47
Diazepam	284.74022 g/mol	2.82	0.8 to 1.0 L/kg [young healthy males]	3.4

Dihydrocodeine	301.38012 g/mol	2.2	The disposition of dihydroco-deine is described as a two compart-ment model.	-
Diluted Tincture of Opium (Paregoric)	Vague data	Vague data	Vague data	Vague data
Disulfiram	296.5392 g/mol	3.88	-	pH of a solution obtained by shaking 1 g with 30 mL of water is 6 to 8
Dronabinol	314.4617 g/mol	6.97	10 L/kg	10.6
Ethanol	46.06844 g/mol	-0.31	-	15.9
Fentanyl	336.47052 g/mol	4.05	3 to 8 L/kg [Surgical Patients] 0.8 to 8 L/kg [Hepatically Impaired Patients]	8.6

Fluoxymesterone	336.440863 g/mol	2.38	-	-
Gamma-hydroxybutyric Acid (GHB)	86.08924 g/mol	-0.64	-	Stable at pH 7
Heroin (diacetylmorphine)	369.41102 g/mol	1.58	-	7.95
Hydrocodone	299.36424 g/mol	1.2	-	8.23
Hydromorphone	285.33766 g/mol	1.8	-	8.9
Khat (Cathinone)	149.18974 g/mol	1.38	-	-
Lysergic Acid Diethylamide (LSD)	323.432 g/mol	2.95	0.28 L/kg	7.8
Marijuana/Cannabis/ Tetrahydro-cannabinol	314.4617 g/mol	5.7	10 L/kg	-

Meperidine	247.33274 g/mol	2.45	3.84 l/kg for therapeutic doses, 5.2 l/kg in cirrhosis of the liver, and 4.5 l/kg in the elderly. Meperidine crosses the placenta and is distributed into breast milk.	8.59
Meprobamate	218.25022 g/mol	0.70	Small volume of distribution (0.7 L/kg)	Aqueous solutions are neutral
Mescaline (Peyote)	211.25758 g/mol	0.78	Not specifically known but is believed to be on the order of several L/kg	9.56
Methadone	309.44518 g/mol	3.93	1.0 to 8.0 L/kg	8.94

Methamphetamine	149.2328 g/mol	2.07	Varies widely, but the average volume of distribution is 5 L/kg	9.87 A saturated solution in water is alkaline to litmus
Methaqualone (Quaalude)	250.29516 g/mol	2.5	Large; 2.4-6.4 l/kg	2.4 Aqueous solution is alkaline to litmus
Methyltestosterone	302.451 g/mol	3.36	-	-
Morphine	285.33766 g/mol	0.89	1 to 6 L/kg	8.21 pH of saturated solution, 8.5
Nalbuphine	357.44338 g/mol	1.4	-	8.71 and 9.96 (HCl form)

Naloxone	327.37434 g/mol	2.09	Following parenteral administration naloxone hydrochloride is rapidly distributed in the body. Naloxone is also very lipophilic and easily crosses the blood-brain-barrier. It can also cross the placenta.	pKa1 = 7.45 (amine); pKa2 = 9.88 (phenol)
Naltrexone	341.40092 g/mol	1.92	1350 L [intravenous administration]	-
Nandrolone	274.39784 g/mol	2.62	-	-
Nicotine	162.23156 g/mol	1.17	2 to 3 L/kg	3.1
Opium	Vague data	Vague data	Vague data	Vague data
Oxandrolone	306.4397 g/mol	2.6	-	-

Oxycodone	315.36364 g/mol	0.66	2.6 L/kg	8.28
Oxymetholone	332.47698 g/mol	4.4	-	-
Oxymorphone	301.33706 g/mol	0.83	3.08 +/- 1.14 L/kg in healthy male and female subjects	8.17
Pentobarbital	226.27222 g/mo	2.10	-	8.11
Phencyclidine	243.3871 g/mol	3.63	Large volume of distribution of 6.2 L/kg	8.29
Phendimetrazine	191.26948 g/mol	1.70	Varies widely	7.3
Propofol	178.27072 g/mol	3.79	60 L/kg [healthy adults]	11.1
Propylhexedrine	155.28044 g/mol	3.5	-	-
Psilocybin	284.248142 g/mol	1.00	-	pH 5.2 in 50% ethanol

Saline Laxatives	-	-	-	-
Secobarbital	238.28292 g/mol	1.97	-	7.8 pH ~ 5.6 saturated solution
Senna Laxatives	862.73912 g/mol	1.2	-	-
Somatrem/Somatropin (Human Growth Hormone)	848.9395 g/mol	-5.2	-	-
Stanozolol	328.49158 g/mol	4.4	-	-
Testolactone	300.39206 g/mol	2.1	-	-
Testosterone	288.42442 g/mol	3.32	-	-
Thiopental	242.33782 g/mol	2.85	0.4-4 L/kg in adults	7.55

*pH is related to pK_a by the Henderson-Hasselbalch pH $= pK_a + \log_{10} ([A^-][HA])$. The ionization constant of a weak acid and original concentration is required to calculate the pH of substances.

**A drug that could be used without medical justification, for its psychoactive effects.

Health care providers should use PubMed and LactMed to manage substance use during breastfeeding. PubChem is a no-cost chemistry database that provides information on biological activities, chemical structures, patents, and more. (8) LactMed is a well-referenced and peer-reviewed online drug breastfeeding database. (9) It is a no-cost resource that can aid healthcare providers to suggest therapeutic alternatives. A table of additional breastfeeding websites is available in "Medications and Breastfeeding: Current Concepts."(1)

The Specifics of Selected Substances

If recreational drugs are used (1), breastfeeding should be interrupted for 24 to 48 hours (24 hours for cocaine) after the last dose. The half-lives for each metabolite may prolong the unsafe duration of the drug. Even with interrupted breastfeeding, infants still may test positive for drugs for days or weeks. Extreme caution should be taken if taking cocaine, LSD, phencyclidine (e.g., angel dust, PCP), hallucinogenic drugs, amphetamines, or IV heroin. PCP and cocaine may be the most dangerous, as the drugs may remain in the baby's system for weeks after the last maternal dose. In addition to the long half-life of the parent drugs, their metabolites have very long half-lives.

Social Considerations

Social considerations related to recreational drug usage include how frequently and how much the mother takes, as well as her ability to care for her baby while under the influence. Mothers on recreational drugs need to be assessed by social services for their dependability. Healthcare professionals should recommend high-risk mothers to discontinue breastfeeding. Low-risk mothers should be given the details of drug transfer into the breast milk and the hazards of the drug to their babies.

Healthcare professionals should let the mother know the hazards of hepatitis B and HIV transfer to the unprotected baby should the mother become infected. Mothers need to know that the baby will test positive during drug screenings for a very long period of time after the mother initially took the drug. There may also be legal consequences of drug screen tests in babies.

Methadone

Questions often arise regarding use of methadone, narcotic pain reliever used to reduce withdrawal symptoms in narcotic addicts, while a mother is breastfeeding. Research has shown that the methadone concentration remains low in the breast milk, such that the potential infant exposure is unlikely to have any negative effect on the developing child. Even at a maximal allowable pediatric dose of 270 micrograms/day, no serious health or developmental concerns have been observed.

When an infant or a pediatric patient needs to be weaned from narcotics, the drug of choice also is methadone. It is given at a low dose of 0.1 mg/Kg/dose every four hours. The half-life in pediatric children is less than adults (children $t_{1/2} = 19 \pm 14$ hours; adult $t_{1/2} = 35 \pm 22$ hours), which means that less exposure to the infant or pediatric patient occurs. Therefore, mothers using methadone are recommended to continue breastfeeding.

Alcohol

Health care professionals often are consulted regarding the use of alcohol. Alcohol rapidly exchanges between the plasma and breast milk. One study has shown that mothers' alcohol use showed a 23% reduction in the amount of milk ingested by babies. The reduced ingestion may be a result of the taste of alcohol in milk. Recent studies suggest that alcohol suppresses oxytocin levels, which reduces milk ejection.

It is more reassuring to know that maternal blood alcohol levels must reach 300 mg [ethanol] in 100 mL blood before affecting the infant considerably. Mothers consuming alcohol can resume breastfeeding after moderate alcohol use as soon as the effects of the alcohol have passed, which is about 1 hour from the end of consumption. Healthcare professionals should also recommend interrupting breastfeeding if the mother consumes more than one drink per hour.

Cigarettes

Cigarette smoke is known to cause a substantial decrease in milk production. Although the exact physiology is unknown, the combination of lower levels of prolactin, elevated somatostatin levels after episodes of suckling, and impaired oxygen delivery and blood flow to the mammary gland may result in lower milk production. As a result, the baby's nursing behavior may change. Also a significant increase of infantile colic has been observed. Milk fat, a crucial component in the baby's development and weight gain, was shown to be at least 19% lower in smoking mothers.

Nicotine cessation therapy should be recommended to smoking mothers, and nicotine replacement therapy, such as nicotine patches or gum, are good as adjuncts to therapy. Nicotine patches with appropriately managed doses were demonstrated to decrease the absolute infant intake of nicotine and its metabolite. Patches not only prevent the rapid entry of nicotine into breast milk, but also reduce the infant's exposure to a cigarette smoke-contaminated environment, and through the mother's metabolism, stop exposure to the direct pharmacologic actions of nicotine, its metabolite, and other toxic substances derived from the cigarette.

Let's Talk

The following questionnaire and approach are published in "Medications and Breastfeeding: Current Concepts."(1) More tips for counseling are provided in Chapter 10.

Questionnaire

During the evaluation of individual patient cases, a health care professional may use the following questions to aid mothers in determining appropriate tactics for making medication therapies more compatible with breastfeeding. This list of questions and step-wise approach are designed for prescription medications. Healthcare providers need to adjust these questions for certain recreational substances based on clinical judgment:

- **What is the name, strength, and dosage form of the drug?** This is the basic information needed to evaluate any situation involving drug use.

- **Do you still have the prescription, or have you already filled it and are taking the drug?** Asking this question helps get the proper perspective regarding the stage of the drug or breastfeeding situation being evaluated. The mother may be seeking advice on whether to continue breastfeeding if and when she takes the drug. She may be questioning whether she is acting correctly by taking the drug and continuing to breastfeed. She also may have concerns about possible adverse effects on her infant.

- **Why is the drug being prescribed?** Discuss with the mother whether the drug is essential in a particular situation. This is best decided with the prescribing physician.

- **Do you feel you need to take the drug?** If the drug is being prescribed for a relatively benign condition, the mother may be willing to endure some personal inconvenience to spare the infant from potential effects of the drug. This also is best decided in conjunction with the prescribing physician.

- **What does your physician say regarding breastfeeding outcome and taking the drug?** A physician's philosophy about breastfeeding and knowledge of drug effects on breastfeeding can play an important role in his/her opinion as to whether the mother should continue to breastfeed. With knowledge of the physician's views on breastfeeding, the mother can decide whether she wants to further pursue the physician's decision. If a physician's philosophy is in conflict with that of the mother, the mother should seek a second opinion.

- **What is the drug dosage schedule and how often do you nurse?** If a drug must be taken by a mother and she wishes to continue to breastfeed, scheduling the doses so that peak plasma and milk levels of the drug do not coincide with breastfeeding sessions may be possible. In most cases, it's best for the mother to breastfeed just before taking a dose of a drug and/or at least two hours after taking a dose. Short-acting drugs taken on an every three-to-six-hour schedule usually reach peak plasma and milk levels in approximately one to two hours.

- **How old is the baby?** The infant's ability to handle a particular drug usually improves with maturity. It also aids in determining the infant's feeding schedule, which may influence dosage scheduling.

- **Was your baby full term or premature?** Premature infants have a reduced ability to detoxify drugs.

- **What is your baby's weight?** This fact may be relevant to the quantity of the drug the baby may be able to tolerate without adverse effects.

- **Is your baby currently receiving any medication**? Any medication that the infant is receiving can interact with medication the infant receives through breast milk.

- **Do you know how to hand express milk or do you have access to a breast pump?** In some cases, breastfeeding can be stopped temporarily while a drug is administered. In these situations, the mother must hand express milk or pump her breasts to prevent breast engorgement and to maintain her milk supply. The mother can learn to hand express milk or to use a breast pump, if necessary, from lactation consultants or La Leche League mothers.

- **Is this your first breastfed baby?** Mothers who have breastfed in the past will be more knowledgeable of the breastfeeding process. A mother who is breastfeeding for the first time may find it more difficult to come to a decision regarding the use of a drug. Involving a lactation consultant in the process, if acceptable to the mother, may be useful.

Stepwise Approach

After a healthcare professional obtains the necessary information to evaluate the patient's case, a safe course of action for the patient should be determined. The following stepwise approach can help patients minimize drug exposure to their newborns:

- **Withhold the drug.** Avoid using nonessential medications by enlisting the mother's cooperation, with the understanding that maintaining maternal health is of paramount importance. Mothers should be advised to use medications only when necessary and important to their health.

- **Try nonpharmacological therapies.** Suggested drug-alternative therapies include analgesics (e.g., relaxation techniques, massage, warm baths); cough, cold, and allergy products (e.g., saline nose drops, cool mist, steam); anti-asthmatic agents (avoid known allergens, particularly animals); antacids (eat small meals, sleep with head propped, avoid head-bending activities, and avoid gas-forming foods); laxatives (eat high-fiber cereal, prunes, or hot liquids with breakfast); antidiarrheal agents (discontinue solids for 12 to 24 hours, increase fluids, eat toast or saltine crackers).

- **Delay therapy.** Mothers who are ready to wean their infant might be able to delay elective drug therapy or elective surgery.

- **Choose drugs that pass poorly into milk.** Large differences in drug distribution into breast milk exist among class members within some drug classes.

- **Choose more breastfeeding–compatible dosage forms.** Take the lowest recommended dose, avoid extra-strength and long-acting preparations, and avoid combination ingredient products.

- **Choose an alternative route of administration.** Local application of drugs to the affected maternal site can minimize drug concentrations in milk and, subsequently, the infant dose.

- **Avoid nursing at times of peak drug concentrations in milk.** Nursing before a dose is given may avoid the peak drug concentrations in milk that occur about one to three hours after an oral dose. This works best for drugs with short half-lives.

- **Administer the drug before the infant's longest sleep period.** This will minimize the infant's dose and is useful for long-acting drugs that can be given once daily.

- **Temporarily withhold breastfeeding.** Depending on the estimated length of drug therapy, nursing can be temporarily withheld. Mothers may be able to pump a sufficient quantity of milk beforehand for use during therapy. The pharmacokinetics of the drug must be examined to determine when the resumption of breastfeeding is advisable.

- **Discontinue nursing.** A few drugs are too toxic to allow nursing and are necessary for the mother's health. Although most drugs appear in breast milk to some degree, the levels usually do not exceed

1% to 2% of ingested maternal dosage. Thus, the amount of drug an infant receives from the mother often is negligible. For example, an infant may receive only about 10 μg (1 microgram = 1 millionth of a gram) when the mother takes 1 mg of a drug or receives 10 ng (1 nanogram = 1 billionth of a gram) when the mother takes 1 μg of the drug. Keeping in mind that the infant has his/her own drug-metabolizing system also is important.

What's New?

Although *Medications and Breastfeeding: Current Concepts* aimed to provide timeless information, new lifestyle concerns now also need to be addressed:

In 2008, the Farm Bill increased research on organic products. (9) The Hartman Group revealed that nearly 60% of U.S. consumers buy organic products, at least occasionally. (10) The organic food and holistic lifestyle movements have grown ever since 2008, evident by the increased accessibility of organic grocery stores.

The Food and Drug Administration (FDA) has initiated a new ruling on pregnancy and lactation labeling to assist healthcare providers in assessing benefits versus risks. This new labeling will need to be incorporated into counseling mothers. (11)

The legalization of small amounts of marijuana use has occurred in Colorado, Washington, Oregon, Alaska, and Washington D.C., with increased acceptance of use in other states; yet the safety of marijuana use is very controversial. (12, 13)

Electronic cigarettes are now very accessible, and their use is highly debated.

Chapter 3: A List of Controlled Substances

Amy C. Luo

Table 3.1 List of Controlled Substances (1-3)

Generic Name	Schedule Class	Legal / Illegal	Drug Class	Labeled Indications
3,4-methylenedioxymeth-amphetamine/MDMA (Ecstasy)	I	I		
3,4-methylenedioxypyro-valeron/MDPV (Bath Salts)	I	I		
Alprazolam	IV	L	Benzodiazepine	Anxiety
Amobarbital	II	L	Barbiturate	Insomnia, Sedation
Amphetamine	II	L	Amphetamine	ADHD, Narcolepsy
Benzphetamine	III	L	Amphetamine	Obesity
Buprenorphine	III	L	Opioid Agonist/ Antagonist	Pain, Opioid dependence
Butalbital	III	L	Barbiturate	Insomnia, Sedation, Headache

Butorphanol	IV	L	Opioid Agonist/ Antagonist	Anesthesia, Pain
Caffeine	RX/OTC	L	Methylxanthine	Headache, Somnolence
Camphor	RX	L	Antitussive, thermal agent	Cough
Carisoprodol	IV	L	Skeletal Muscle Relaxant: Centrally Acting	Disorder of musculoskele-tal system
Chloral Hydrate	IV	L	Nonbarbiturate Hypnotic	Insomnia, Sedation
Chlordiazepoxide	IV	L	Benzodiazepine	Alcohol Withdrawal Syndrome, Anxiety
Cocaine	I	I	Stimulant	Non-FDA: Cluster headache
Cocaine (Topical)	II		Anesthetic	Non-FDA: Local anesthesia
Codeine	II	L	Opioid	Pain
Cyclobenzaprine	RX	L	Skeletal Muscle Relaxant: Centrally Acting	Skeletal muscle spasm
Dextroamphetamine	II	L	Amphetamine	ADHD, Narcolepsy
Diazepam	IV	L	Benzodiazepine	Alcohol Withdrawal Syndrome, Anxiety, Sedation, Seizures

Dihydrocodeine	II	L	Opioid	Heart failure, Postoperative pain, Pulmonary emphysema
Diluted Tincture of Opium (Paregoric)	III	L	Opioid	Diarrhea
Disulfiram	RX	L	Dependency Agent	Alcoholism
Dronabinol	III	L	Cannabinoid	AIDS - Loss of appetite, Chemotherapy-induced nausea and vomiting
Ethanol	RX/ OTC	L		Ethylene glycol toxicity, Methanol toxicity
Fentanyl	II	L	Opioid	Anesthesia, Pain
Fluoxymesterone	III	L	Androgen	Breast cancer, Palliative treatment, Delayed puberty, Hypogonado-tropic hypogonadism, Primary hypogonadism
Gamma-hydroxybutyric Acid (GHB)	I			
Heroin (diacetylmorphine)	I		Opioid	Opioid abuse, Pain

Hydrocodone	II	L	Opioid	Pain
Hydromorphone	II	L	Opioid	Pain
Ketamine	III	L	Anesthetic	Anesthesia, Sedation
Khat (Cathinone)	I		Stimulant	Non-FDA: Cognitive functioning (inconclusive data), Psychological functioning (ineffective), Reproductive toxicity
Lysergic Acid Diethylamide (LSD)	I			
Marijuana/Cannabis /Tetrahydro-cannabinol	I		Cannabinoid	
Meperidine	II	L	Opioid	Anesthesia, Pain
Meprobamate	IV	L	Carbamate, Anti-anxiety	Anxiety
Mescaline (Peyote)	I			
Methadone	II	L	Opioid	Drug detoxification - Opioid abuse, Pain
Methamphetamine	II	L	Amphetamine	ADHD, Obesity
Methaqualone (Quaalude)	I		Sedative-hypnotic	Insomnia

Methylphenidate	II	L	Amphetamine Related - CNS Stimulant	ADHD, Narcolepsy
Methyltestosterone	III	L	Androgen	Delay in sexual development AND/OR puberty (Male), Hypogonado-tropic hypogonadism, Metastasis from malignant tumor of breast, inoperable metastatic disease (skeletal) in women 1 to 5 years postmenopau-sal, Primary hypogonadism
Morphine	II	L	Opioid	Pain
Nalbuphine	RX	L	Opioid	Anesthesia, Pain
Naloxone	RX	L	Opioid Antagonist	Opiate overdose
Naltrexone	RX	L	Opioid Antagonist	Alcohol dependence, Opioid dependence

Nandrolone	III	L	Anabolic Steroid, Androgen	Anemia
Nicotine	RX/OTC	L		
Opium	I		Opioid	
Oxandrolone	III	L	Anabolic Steroid	Weight gain
Oxycodone	II	L	Opioid	Pain
Oxymetholone	III	L	Androgen	Acquired aplastic anemia, Anemia of chronic renal failure, Antineoplastic adverse reaction – Myelosuppression, Fanconi's anemia, Pure red cell aplasia
Oxymorphone	II	L	Opioid	Anesthesia, Anxiety, Pain
Pentazocine	IV	L	Opioid Agonist/ Antagonist	Anesthesia, Pain.
Pentobarbital	II or III (based on route, form, strength	L	Barbiturate	Anesthesia, Insomnia, Sedation, Seizures
Phencyclidine	I		Hallucinogen	
Phendimetrazine	III	L	Amphetamine Related	Obesity

Propofol	RX	L	Sedative-hypnotic	Anesthesia, Sedation
Propylhexedrine	OTC	L	Amphetamine Related	Nasal congestion
Psilocybin	I		Hallucinogen	
Saline Laxatives	OTC			
Secobarbital	II	L	Barbiturate	Anesthesia, Insomnia
Senna Laxatives	OTC			
Somatrem/Somatropin (Human Growth Hormone)	RX	L	Pituitary hormone	Growth hormone deficiency, Decreased body growth - Prader-Willi Syndrome, Noonan's Syndrome - Short stature disorder, Renal function impairment with growth failure, Small for gestational age baby, with no catch-up growth by age 2 to 4 years

Stanozolol	III	L	Anabolic Steroid	Antithrombin III deficiency, Cryofibrinogenemia, Hereditary angiodemia, Lichen sclerosus et atrophicus, Lipodermato-sclerosis, Protein C deficiency disease, Raynaud's phenomenon, Rheumatoid arthritis, Thrombosis, Urticaria
Testolactone	III	L	Androgen	Breast cancer, Advanced or disseminated disease (as adjunct therapy during palliative treatment)
Testosterone	III	L	Androgen	Primary hypogonadism (Male) Delayed puberty (Male) Metastatic breast cancer (Female)

Thiopental	III	L	Barbiturate	Anesthesia, Narcoanalysis, Raised intracranial pressure, Seizures

Substances by Class (4)

Amphetamines / Stimulants

In dosages prescribed for medical indications, some evidence indicates that amphetamines do not affect nursing infants adversely. The effect of amphetamines in milk on the neurological development of the infant has not been well studied. Large dosages of amphetamines might interfere with milk production, especially in women whose lactation is not well established. Breastfeeding is generally discouraged in mothers who are actively abusing amphetamines.

Anabolic Steroids

There are no data on the excretion of anabolic steroids into human milk. Because many drugs are excreted into human milk and because of the potential for adverse effects on the nursing infant, a decision should be made to discontinue nursing or discontinue the drug, taking into account the importance of the drug to the woman.

Androgens

Limited data indicate that a low-dose (100 mg) subcutaneous testosterone pellet given to a nursing mother appears not to increase milk testosterone levels markedly. Testosterone has low oral bioavailability because of extensive first-pass metabolism, so it is unlikely to affect the breastfed infant. One breastfed infant seemed not to be adversely affected by low-dose maternal testosterone therapy.

There are no data on the excretion of other androgens listed in the table above. Because many drugs are excreted into human milk and because of the potential for adverse effects on the nursing infant, a decision should be made to discontinue nursing or discontinue the drug, taking into account the importance of the drug to the woman.

Barbiturates / Nonbarbiturates Hypnotics

Inter- and intrapatient variability in excretion of phenobarbital into breast milk is extensive. Phenobarbital in breast milk apparently can decrease

50

withdrawal symptoms in infants who were exposed in utero, but it can also cause drowsiness in some infants, especially when used with other sedating drugs. Monitor the infant for drowsiness, adequate weight gain, and developmental milestones, especially in younger, exclusively breastfed infants and when using combinations of psychotropic drugs. Sometimes breastfeeding might have to be limited or discontinued because of excessive drowsiness and poor weight gain. If there is concern, measurement of the infant's serum phenobarbital concentration might help rule out toxicity.

There is little published experience with other barbiturates during breastfeeding, thus other agents may be preferred, especially while nursing a newborn or preterm infant.

Benzodiazepines

The "LOT" group of benzodiazepines has short half-lives relative to other benzodiazepines. Lorazepam (L) and oxazepam (O) can safely be administered directly to infants, and temazepam (T) has low levels in breast milk. These benzodiazepines would not be expected to cause any adverse effects in breastfed infants with usual maternal dosages. No special precautions are required.

Midazolam also exists in small quantity in breast milk. However, an active metabolite can accumulate in the mother and might affect the infant, but data in breastfeeding are lacking.

There is little to no published experience with flurazepam, triazolam, and quazepam during breastfeeding, thus other agents may be preferred, especially while nursing a newborn or preterm infant.

Lastly, due to reports of effects in infants, including sedation, alprazolam is probably not the best benzodiazepine for repeated use during nursing, especially with a neonate or premature infant. A shorter-acting benzodiazepine without active metabolites is preferred. After a single dose of alprazolam, there is usually no need to wait to resume breastfeeding.

Cannabinoids

Although published data are limited, it appears that active components of marijuana are excreted into breast milk in small quantities (5). Data are from random breast milk screening rather than controlled studies because of ethical considerations in administering marijuana to nursing mothers. Concern has been expressed regarding marijuana's possible effects on neurotransmitters, nervous system development, and endocannabinoid-related functions. One long-term study found that daily or near daily use might retard the breastfed infant's motor development, but not growth or intellectual development. This and another study found that occasional maternal marijuana use during breastfeeding did not have any discernible effects on breastfed infants, but the studies were inadequate to rule out all long-term harm. Although marijuana can affect serum prolactin variably, it appears not to adversely affect the duration of lactation. Other factors to consider are the possibility of positive urine tests in breastfed infants, which might have legal implications, and the possibility of other harmful contaminants in street drugs. Health professionals' opinions on the acceptability of breastfeeding by marijuana-using mothers vary considerably.

Marijuana use should be minimized or avoided by nursing mothers because it may impair their judgment and child-care abilities. Some evidence indicates that paternal marijuana use increases the risk of sudden infant death syndrome in breastfed infants. Marijuana should not be smoked by anyone in the vicinity of infants because the infants may be exposed by inhaling the smoke. Because breastfeeding can mitigate some of the effects of smoking and little evidence of serious infant harm has been seen, it appears preferable to encourage mothers who use marijuana to continue breastfeeding and reducing or abstaining from marijuana use while minimizing infant exposure to marijuana smoke.

Dronabinol (**tetrahydrocannabinol**) is a major active component of cannabis. As a pharmaceutical product, it has not been studied during breastfeeding, but limited data from marijuana smokers indicate that it is likely excreted into breast milk and found in the urine of breastfed infants. Concern has been expressed regarding marijuana's possible effects on neurotransmitters, nervous system development, and endocannabinoid-related functions. Studies in marijuana smokers have had contradictory findings. One long-term study found that daily or near daily use might retard the breastfed infant's motor development, but not growth or intellectual development. This and another study found that occasional maternal marijuana use during breastfeeding did not have any discernible effects on breastfed infants, but the studies were inadequate to rule out all long-term harm.

Because there is no published experience with dronabinol use as an antiemetic during breastfeeding, an alternate drug may be preferred, especially while nursing a newborn or preterm infant.

Hallucinogens

A single case of phencyclidine use has been reported in which a small amount of phencyclidine was detected in breast milk over six weeks after use of an unknown quantity of the drug. Effects on the breastfed infant are unknown.

The Academy of Breastfeeding Medicine (ABM) suggests that women who have abused phencyclidine generally should not breastfeed unless they have a negative maternal urine toxicology at delivery, have been abstinent for at least 90 days, are in a substance abuse treatment program and plan to continue in it during the postpartum period, have the approval of their substance abuse counselor, have been engaged and compliant in their prenatal care, and have no other contraindications to breastfeeding.

Methylxanthine Stimulants

Caffeine appears in breast milk rapidly after maternal ingestion. Fussiness, jitteriness, and poor sleep patterns have been reported in the infants of mothers with very high caffeine intakes equivalent to about 10 or more cups of coffee daily. Studies in mothers taking five cups of coffee daily found no stimulatory effects on infants three weeks of age and older. Some experts feel that a maternal intake limit of 300 mg daily might be a safe level of intake. However, preterm and younger newborn infants metabolize caffeine very slowly and may have serum levels of caffeine and other active caffeine metabolites similar to their mothers' levels, so a lower intake level is preferable in the mothers of these infants. Other sources of caffeine, such as cola and energy drinks, yerba mate, or guarana, will have similar dose-related effects on the breastfed infant. Coffee intake of more than 450 mL daily may decrease breast milk iron concentrations and result in mild iron deficiency anemia in some breastfed infants.

Opioids / Opioid-Agonists / Antagonists

Most maternal use of oral narcotics during breastfeeding can cause infant drowsiness, central nervous system depression and even death. Newborn infants seem to be particularly sensitive to the effects of even small dosages of narcotic analgesics. Once the mother's milk comes in, it is best to provide pain control with a nonnarcotic analgesic and limit maternal intake of most opioid analgesics with close infant monitoring. If the baby shows signs of increased sleepiness (more than usual), difficulty breastfeeding, breathing difficulties, or limpness, a physician should be contacted immediately.

Exceptions include buprenorphine, nalbuphine, fentanyl, and methadone.

Due to the low levels of **buprenorphine** in breast milk, its poor oral bioavailability in infants, and the low drug concentrations found in the serum and urine of breastfed infants, its use is acceptable in nursing mothers. Women who received buprenorphine for opiate abuse during pregnancy and are stable should be encouraged to breastfeed their infants postpartum, unless there is another contraindication, such as use of street drugs. The breastfeeding rate among mothers taking buprenorphine for opiate addiction may be lower than in other mothers.

Nalbuphine is excreted into breast milk in amounts much smaller than the dose given to infants for analgesia. Because nalbuphine has poor oral absorption, it is unlikely to adversely affect the breastfed infant. No special precautions are required. Labor pain medication may delay the onset of lactation.

When used epidurally or intravenously during labor or for a short time immediately postpartum, amounts of **fentanyl** ingested by the neonate are small and are not expected to cause any adverse effects in breastfed infants. No waiting period or discarding of milk is required before resuming breastfeeding after fentanyl is used for short procedures (e.g., for endoscopy). After general anesthesia, breastfeeding can be resumed as soon as the mother has recovered sufficiently from anesthesia to nurse. When a combination of anesthetic agents is used for a procedure, follow the recommendations for the most problematic medication used during the procedure. Limited information indicates that transdermal fentanyl in a dosage of 100 mcg/hour results in undetectable fentanyl concentrations in breast milk.

Most infants receive an estimated dose of **methadone** ranging from 1% to 3% of the mother's weight-adjusted methadone dosage with a few receiving 5% to 6%, which is less than the dosage used for treating neonatal abstinence. Initiation of methadone postpartum, increasing the maternal dosage to greater than 100 mg daily therapeutically, or by abuse while breastfeeding poses a risk of sedation and respiratory depression in the breastfed infant, especially if the infant was not exposed to methadone in utero. If the baby shows signs of increased sleepiness (more than usual), breathing difficulties, or limpness, a physician should be contacted immediately. Other agents are preferred over methadone for pain control during breastfeeding.

Women who received methadone maintenance during pregnancy and are stable should be encouraged to breastfeed their infants postpartum, unless there is another contraindication, such as use of street drugs. Breastfeeding may decrease, but not eliminate, neonatal withdrawal symptoms in infants who were exposed in utero. Some studies have found shorter hospital stays, shorter durations of neonatal abstinence therapy, and shorter durations of therapy among breastfed infants, although the dosage of opiates used for neonatal abstinence may not be reduced. Abrupt weaning of breastfed

54

infants of women on methadone maintenance might result in precipitation of or an increase in infant withdrawal symptoms, and gradual weaning is advised. The breastfeeding rate among mothers taking methadone for opiate addiction has been lower than in mothers not using methadone in some studies, but this finding appears to vary by institution, indicating that other factors may be important.

Pituitary Hormones

No information is available on the clinical use of corticotropin during breastfeeding. It is unlikely to appear in breast milk because it is has a molecular weight (mass) of 4,540 and a half-life of only 10 to 15 minutes. Absorption by the infant is unlikely because it would probably be destroyed in the infant's gastrointestinal tract. Based on animal data, an increase in breast milk cortisol levels might be expected after administration of corticotropin to a nursing mother. If corticotropin is required by the mother, it is not a reason to discontinue breastfeeding.

Sedatives / Hypnotics

Short-term or occasional use of chloral hydrate during breastfeeding is unlikely to adversely affect the breastfed infant, especially if the infant is older than two months. Because the active metabolite of chloral hydrate has a long half-life, other sedative-hypnotics are preferred for long-term use during breastfeeding, especially while nursing a neonate or preterm infant. Monitor the infant for excessive drowsiness.

The list above is not a comprehensive list of controlled substances that have the potential to be used during pregnancy or breastfeeding.

Chapter 4: Review of ABM Protocol #21 and List of Breastfeeding Questions for Healthcare Professionals

Amy C. Luo

I was fielding calls from our volunteer nursing mothers' group warmline and got a call from a worried mother. She'd taken Ecstasy the day before, and was wondering about nursing her 6-week-old baby.

At that time, there wasn't anything published about this. I advised waiting 24 hours after the last flashback (pumping and dumping) before nursing again. She was distraught and I validated her distress! I also praised her for calling for help. What a crazy thing to do.

I have no way of knowing what she actually did.

(Name withheld by request; used with permission)

Introduction

The Academy of Breastfeeding Medicine (ABM) is a worldwide organization of physicians dedicated to the promotion, protection, and support of breastfeeding and human lactation.

The ABM Protocol Committee published *Clinical Protocol #21: Guidelines for Breastfeeding and the Drug-Dependent Woman* in 2009, and then *Clinical Protocol #21: Guidelines for Breastfeeding and Substance Use or Substance Use Disorder, Revised 2015* in Volume 10, Number 3, 2015 of the Breastfeeding Medicine Journal.

Several changes from 2009 to the revised 2015 guideline include: (1, 2)

- Data from two studies published in 2011 and 2013
- In depth discussion of methadone, buprenorphine, and marijuana/tetrahydrocannabinol (THC)
- Considerations for alcohol and tobacco use
- Online websites with updated breastfeeding and drug information
- Substance and substance class specific recommendations

Both the U.K. study published in 2011 and the Norwegian study published in 2013 showed lower rates of breastfeeding initiation in mothers who used illicit substances or were on opioid therapy during pregnancy. Mothers may believe that they should not breastfeed with drug use, they may have impaired decision making due to illicit substance use, and they may also be unaware of the benefits of breastfeeding.

Protocol

The protocol provides guidance in managing common medical problems that may impact breastfeeding success. It describes the relevance of recreational drug use in the breastfeeding population. Specific substances discussed include methadone, buprenorphine, opioids as a drug class, marijuana, alcohol, and tobacco. The protocol also provides current recommendations for physicians to implement individual care plans and suggests future research topics.

When healthcare providers are implementing Protocol #21, note that:

Patient outreach and education is of utmost importance. Patients can easily misinterpret the explanation of "drugs of any type should be avoided in pregnant and breastfeeding women, unless prescribed for specific medical conditions" as "drug use = do not breastfeed." It is up to the healthcare provider and healthcare worker to tailor this statement to individual patient cases.

Methadone is the treatment of choice for pregnant and postpartum women with opioid dependence. However, the lack of primary care providers, limited access to healthcare facilities, and the negative perception of maternal methadone use by healthcare providers and workers create challenges for substance-dependent mothers to seek help.

Protocol #21 "serves only as guidelines for the care of breastfeeding mothers and infants and does not delineate an exclusive course of treatment or serve as standards of medical care." Online websites listed in Protocol #21 can aid healthcare providers make informed clinical judgments:

- LactMed (English): http://toxnet.nlm.nih.gov/cgi-bin/sis/htmlgen?LACT
- e-Lactancia (English/Spanish): www.e-lactancia.org

Summary

The Baby-Friendly Hospital Initiative (BFHI) encourages and recognizes hospitals and birthing centers that offer an "optimal level of care for infant feeding and mother/baby bonding." (3) BFHI is an initiative launched by the World Health Organization (WHO) and the United Nations Children's Fund (UNICEF) that requires training and skill building among all levels of staff. ABM is historically comprised of physicians only. Since nurses, pharmacists, and other healthcare professionals are crucial in making BFHI a success, Protocol #21 can benefit from collaboration with a multidisciplinary team.

Prior to the availability of the ABM protocol #21, healthcare providers lacked standardized guidance. ABM states that their protocols "expire five (5) years from the date of publication." Evidence-based revisions are made "within five (5) years or sooner if there are significant changes in the evidence." Although it is difficult to collect and draw conclusions from a limited sample, Protocol #21 complements issues discussed in this book and shall continually be updated as data become available.

List of Questions to Ask in Breastfeeding / Medication Situations

Over many years of practice and experience while working with mothers, families, and healthcare professionals, the primary author developed a list of questions to ask in breastfeeding /medication situations. These questions can be used by a multidisciplinary team to complement the standardized guidance provided by ABM Clinical Protocol #21 and as part of the Baby-Friendly Hospital Initiative. The questions can be asked by any healthcare professional, especially pharmacists, involved in the breastfeeding process, as needed and as necessary. The questions can be adapted to ask regarding, not only prescription drug use, but also Over-the-Counter (OTC), herbal, supplemental drug, social, recreational, illegal, and any other conceivable drug use. The List of Questions to Ask in Breastfeeding / Medication Situations and the rationale for each of the questions is found in Appendix 5.

Chapter 5: Schedule I Drugs

I have personal experience with smoking marijuana while breastfeeding. All my breastfeeding experience was before becoming an IBCLC, and I breastfed my three children for an average of three years each. I smoked marijuana once every several months during breastfeeding. I never took any precaution to separate drug use and breastfeeding (aside from not smoking while breastfeeding), and I never noticed any adverse reaction in my children. What I worried about the most was what I would do in an emergency situation, which did not happen, but there was no way to know that in advance.

(Name withheld by request; used with permission)

Introduction

Schedule I drugs have a high potential for abuse. These drugs have no currently accepted medical use in disease or disorders treatment. There is also a lack of accepted safety for use of these drugs under medical supervision. If these drugs are used, it is usually for nonhuman research. Tetrahydrocannabinol (THC)/marijuana under current federal law is considered a Schedule I drug by the Drug Enforcement Agency (DEA) (1, 2), even though some states have "legalized" it for recreation or medical use. Marijuana will be covered specifically in Chapter 6. Schedule I drugs should always be contraindicated for use by pregnant and breastfeeding women. This is very obvious when one notes the extreme negative health risks associated with each substance of abuse. (3) In addition, drug abusers commonly use multiple drugs, including tobacco and especially alcohol. The following are those drugs that have the potential for abuse by pregnant and/or breastfeeding women and potential disastrous effects on the unborn and breastfeeding child. (4)

Schedule I Drugs

Cocaine: Cocaine is a powerful addictive stimulant drug made from the leaves of the South American coca plant. Cocaine is one of the most dangerous drugs of abuse. (5) Drug abuse can lead to tachycardia (rapid heart rate), tachypnea (rapid breathing), hypertension, irritability, and tremulousness in abusers and in breastfed children of abusers. Other short-term and long-term health effects include narrowed blood vessels, enlarged pupils, increased body temperature, headache, abdominal pain, nausea, euphoria, insomnia, restlessness, anxiety, erratic and violent behavior, panic attacks, paranoia, psychosis, heart attack, stroke, seizures, coma, loss of smell, nosebleeds, damaged swallowing, infection, necrosis of bowel tissue, poor nutrition, and weight loss. Of special interest for pregnancy are spontaneous abortion in early pregnancy, premature delivery, low birth rate, stillbirth, congenital abnormalities (brain and cardiac), and Neonatal Abstinence Syndrome (see Chapter 8). The pregnant mother is at risk for HIV, hepatitis, and other infectious diseases from shared needle use. Significant cognitive deficits have occurred in cocaine-exposed children through pregnancy. Cocaine rapidly crosses the placental barrier, and higher concentrations occur in the fetus. Children after birth are twice as likely to have significant delay for the first two years of life, although other studies show no difference at four years of age. Mental retardation rates are almost five times as high as the normal population. At the same time, the rate for mild or greater delays requiring intervention is twice as much. There is a case report of a breastfed infant having apnea (suspension of breathing) and seizures after ingesting cocaine applied to the nipple as an anesthetic. In combination with alcohol, there is a greater risk of overdose and sudden death than from either drug alone.

Gamma-hydroxybutyric Acid (GHB): GHB is not to be confused with sodium oxybate, a drug used to treat narcolepsy. GHB is used illegally to produce euphoria, disinhibition, enhanced sensuality, and to induce empathy and sympathy. Side effects include euphoria, drowsiness, decreased anxiety, confusion, memory loss, hallucinations, excited and aggressive behavior, nausea, vomiting, unconsciousness, seizures, slowed heart rate and breathing, lower body temperatures, coma, and death. In combination with alcohol, there is a greater risk of nausea, problems with breathing, and greatly increased depressant effects.

Heroin: Heroin is an opioid drug made from morphine, a natural substance extracted from the seed pod of the Asian opium poppy plant. Health risks include euphoria, warm flushing of the skin, dry mouth, heavy feeling in hands and feet, unclear thinking processes, alternating states of wakefulness and drowsiness, itching, nausea, vomiting, slowed breathing and heart rates, collapsed veins, abscesses, heart lining and valve infections, constipation, stomach cramps, liver or kidney disease, pneumonia, and death. Heroin is the most commonly abused opioid, and it crosses the placental barrier and enters fetal tissues within one hour of maternal use. Heroin users are usually multi-substance abusers, which potentiates adverse effects. Especially relevant for pregnant women is miscarriage, low birth rate, and Neonatal Abstinence

Syndrome (see Chapter 8). There is also the risk for HIV, hepatitis, and other infectious disease from shared needle use. There can be severe consequences for the fetus and newborn for fetal development disorders or Sudden Infant Death Syndrome (SIDS). In combination with alcohol, there is a greater risk of a dangerous slowdown of heart rate and breathing, coma, and death.

Lysergic Acid Diethylamide (LSD): LSD is a hallucinogen manufactured from lysergic acid, which is found in ergot, a fungus that grows on rye and other grains. Health effects include rapid emotional swings; distortion of the ability to recognize reality, think rationally, or communicate with others; hypertension; increased heart rate; increased body temperature; dizziness; insomnia; loss of appetite; dry mouth; sweating; numbness; weakness; tremors; enlarged pupils; frightening flashbacks (sudden vivid memory); ongoing visual disturbances; disorganized thinking; paranoia; and mood swings. In combination with alcohol, there may be a decreased perception of the effects of alcohol.

Marijuana / Cannabis / Tetrahydrocannabinol: Marijuana is made from the hemp plant. The main psychoactive (mind altering) chemical in marijuana is delta-9-tetrahydrocannabinol or THC. Due to the unique status of being used at state levels "legally" and/or medically, marijuana will be discussed in a separate chapter (see Chapter 6).

Mescaline (Peyote): Mescaline, also known as peyote, is a hallucinogen found in disk-shaped buttons in the crown of several cacti, including peyote. Health effects include enhanced perception and feeling, hallucinations, euphoria, anxiety, increased body temperature, increased heart rate, hypertension, sweating, movement problems, and unknown long-term effects. The effects of simultaneous alcohol consumption are unknown.

Methaqualone (Quaalude): Methaqualone is a central nervous system (CNS) depressant of the quinazolinone class of drug substances that acts as a sedative and hypnotic. When the primary author was first practicing as a pharmacist in the 1960s, methaqualone use peaked as a hypnotic for the treatment of insomnia, as a sedative, and as a muscle relaxant. As it was replaced by prescription drug products with less abuse potential and deleterious side effects, it was and is still produced and used illegally as a recreational drug worldwide. Health related effects include drowsiness, reduced heart rate, reduced respiration, increased sexual arousal (aphrodisia), and paresthesias (numbness of the fingers and toes). Larger doses can lead to respiratory depression, slurred speech, headache, and photophobia (a symptom of excessive sensitivity to light). Overdoses can cause delirium, convulsions, hypertonia (abnormal increase in muscle tension and a reduced ability of a muscle to stretch), hyperreflexia (overactive or over-responsive reflexes), vomiting, kidney failure, coma, and death (cardiac or respiratory arrest). It resembles barbiturate poisoning, but with increased motor difficulties and a lower incidence of cardiac or respiratory depression. Combining alcohol greatly potentiates the effects of methaqualone.

3, 4-methylenedioxymethamphetamine / MDMA (Ecstasy): MDMA, also known as Ecstasy, is a synthetic, psychoactive drug that has similarities to both amphetamines (stimulants) and to mescaline (hallucinogen). Negative health effects include lowered inhibition; enhanced sensory perception; confusion; depression; sleep problems; anxiety, increased heart rate; hypertension; muscle tension; teeth clenching; nausea; blurred vision; faintness; chills or sweating; sharp rises in body temperature leading to liver, kidney, or heart failure; long lasting confusion; depression; attention, memory, and sleep problems; impulsiveness; aggression; loss of appetite; and less interest in sex. In combination with alcohol, there is a greater risk of cell and organ damage.

3,4-methylenedioxypyrovalerone / MDPV (Bath Salts): Bath salts are an emerging family of drugs containing one or more synthetic chemicals related to Cathinone, a stimulant found in the Khat plant (leaves of the shrub are typically chewed and held in the cheek, like chewing tobacco, to release their stimulant chemicals). Examples of these chemicals include mephedrone, methylone, and 3, 4-methylenedioxypyrovalerone. Health effects include increased heart rate, hypertension, euphoria, increased sociability and sex drive, paranoia, agitation, hallucinations, psychotic and violent behavior, nosebleeds, sweating, nausea, vomiting, insomnia, irritability, dizziness, depression, suicidal thoughts, panic attacks, reduced motor control, unclear thinking, breakdown of skeletal muscle tissue, kidney failure, and death. The effects of using alcohol at the same time with bath salts are unknown.

Opium: Opium is a highly addictive narcotic drug acquired in the dried latex form from the opium poppy seed pod. Traditionally the unripened pod is slit open, and the sap seeps out and dries on the outer surface of the pod. The resulting yellow-brown latex, which is scraped off of the pod, is bitter in taste and contains varying amounts of alkaloids, such as morphine, codeine, thebaine, and papaverine. Opium effects include drowsiness, nausea, constipation, euphoria, confusion, slowed breathing, and death. Pregnancy issues include miscarriage, low birth weight, and Neonatal Abstinence Syndrome (NAS) (see Chapter 8). Pregnant mothers are at risk for HIV, hepatitis, and other infectious diseases from shared needle use. There can be severe consequences for the fetus and newborn for fetal development disorders or Sudden Infant Death Syndrome (SIDS). In combination with alcohol, there is a higher risk of dangerous slowing of the heart rate and breathing leading to coma or death.

Phencyclidine (PCP): Phencyclidine is a potent hallucinogen that has long half-life metabolites. It is one of the most dangerous of all drugs of abuse. Phencyclidine is commonly known as PCP and Angel Dust. A number of synthetic derivatives of PCP have been sold as hallucinogenic drugs for recreational and nonmedical use. The list of deleterious health risks is voluminous and includes feelings of being detached, distant, and estranged from surroundings; numbness of extremities; slurred speech; and loss of coordination accompanied by a sense of strength and invulnerability; blank stares; rapid and involuntary eye movements; exaggerated gait; auditory hallucinations; image distortion; severe mood disorders; amnesia; acute anxiety; feelings of impending doom; paranoia; violent hostility, psychosis indistinguishable from schizophrenia; increased breathing rate; pronounced rises in blood pressure and pulse rate; shallow respiration; flushing; and profuse sweating. At high doses of phencyclidine, there is a drop in blood pressure, pulse rate, and respiration. This may be accompanied by nausea, vomiting, blurred vision, flicking up and down of the eyes, drooling, loss of balance, and dizziness. High doses of phencyclidine can also cause seizures, coma, and death (though death more often results from accidental injury or suicide during phencyclidine intoxication). Psychological effects at high doses include illusions and hallucinations. Phencyclidine is addictive and its use often leads to psychological dependence, craving, and compulsive phencyclidine-seeking behavior. Users of phencyclidine report memory loss, difficulties with speech and learning, depression, and weight loss. These symptoms can persist up to a year after cessation of phencyclidine use. In combination with alcohol, there is an increased risk of coma.

Psilocybin: Psilocybin is a hallucinogen from certain types of mushrooms from South America, Mexico, and the United States. Health side effects include hallucinations, altered perceptions of time, inability to tell fantasy from reality, panic, muscle relaxation or weakness, movement problems, enlarged pupils, nausea, vomiting, drowsiness, risks of flashbacks, memory problems, and poisoning and death if poisonous mushrooms are accidently used. Using alcohol also may decrease the perceived effects of the alcohol.

Chapter 6: Marijuana

Frank J. Nice

Interview questions for and responses from a mother who used marijuana while breastfeeding:

1. Why did you decide to use marijuana while breastfeeding, i.e., for fun, for relaxation, for self-medicating purposes (i.e., pain or anxiety)?

    I used marijuana while breastfeeding in order to help manage my postpartum depression and anxiety. I had also used it during pregnancy to curb my nausea, which allowed me to eat and gain a healthy amount of weight.

2. Did you have any concerns about using marijuana while breastfeeding? If so, what were they?

    If at all, I was worried about the stigma that simply accompanies smoking marijuana, let alone while pregnant.

3. How did you feel about your decision, i.e., did you feel comfortable, did you have concerns but felt that the benefits outweighed the risks?

    I felt, and still feel completely comfortable with my decision. I was able to avoid taking any pharmaceutical drugs and, therefore, did not have to manage their side effects or put my breastfeeding relationship in jeopardy.

4. Why did you decide to continue breastfeeding and using marijuana at the same time?

    I needed a way to manage my postpartum depression and anxiety and did not want to suffer from the risks and side effects of pharmaceuticals. It also helped my appetite, which was important, as I needed to ingest even more calories while breastfeeding.

5. Were you aware of current (though admittedly lacking) research based on marijuana and breastfeeding?

    Yes, and I was also aware of research done (or not done) surrounding anti-anxiety and antidepressant medications on lactating mothers and their children and the side effects that accompany them. I made the choice that was best for me that allowed me to have maximum benefits with minimal side effects.

6. What adverse effects had you heard / read about?

> I do not recall what I have read specifically about marijuana and breastfeeding and adverse effects, aside from the line that "your child will be slower to develop", which I will constantly disagree with. One adverse effect that I have experienced is that it is dehydrating, which can cause issues for a lactating mother who is not ensuring that she stay well hydrated.

7. Did you separate intake of marijuana and breastfeeding by a certain amount of time? If so, what amount of time, and if not, why not?

> Ideally I would nurse my little one down to sleep and then smoke. If that was not possible, I would prefer to breastfeed and then use marijuana.

8. Did you use any cleansing techniques to rid your body of marijuana? If so, how did you hear about this technique?

> No, I did not hear of anything specific to cleanse; however, I do take Epsom salt baths, which I assume would be cleansing.

9. Did you notice your infant being affected by the use of this drug? If so, what effects were observed?

> No, not at all.

(Name withheld by request; used with permission)

Marijuana Introduction

Marijuana (Cannabis): Marijuana is made from the hemp plant, Cannabis sativa. (1) The main psychoactive (mind-altering) chemical in marijuana is delta-9-tetrahydrocannabinol, or THC. Health effects of marijuana include enhanced sensory perception and euphoria followed by drowsiness and relaxation, slowed reaction times, problems with balance and coordination, increased heart rate and appetite, problems with learning and memory, hallucinations, anxiety, panic attacks, psychosis, mental health problems, chronic cough, and frequent respiratory infections. (2-6) Combination with alcohol results in increased heart rate, hypertension, and further slowing of mental processes and reaction time. When one reads these negative health effects, one can see why marijuana is classified as a Schedule I substance of abuse. Many of these effects have been determined with a high level of confidence. Addiction to marijuana is real, as approximately 9% of those who experiment with marijuana become addicted, which increases to 17% of adolescents. One-half of those who smoke daily become addicted. This is shown by a cannabis withdrawal syndrome that includes irritability, insomnia, dysphoria (state of unease or generalized dissatisfaction with life), and anxiety. Societal implications go beyond these clinical implications, such as poor school performance, dropping out of school, lower intelligence scores, unemployment, criminal behavior, lower income, reduced satisfaction with life, increased motor vehicle accidents, and increased risk of using other illicit drugs.

Apparent negative health results during pregnancy include babies born with attention problems, memory problems, and problem solving issues. (7-9) Several studies have shown no increased risk for miscarriage rates, types of presentation at birth, Apgar status, neonatal complications, or major physical abnormalities, although heavy users reported true ocular hypertelorism (increased distance between the eyes) and severe epicanthus (a vertical fold of skin on either side of the nose). The reality is that the small number of studies has failed to identify major birth defects, while at the same time it is a fact that marijuana does cross the placental barrier. As for breastfeeding babies, any kind of smoke is a health risk. THC passes from the mother's plasma into breast milk. Breastfed babies can have problems with feeding and development, both mentally and physically. When the authors reviewed the numerous potential health problems induced by marijuana in adults, it is hard to conclude that unborn and breastfeeding children would be innocuous to them. Schedule I drug substances, which of course include marijuana, have a high potential for abuses, have no currently accepted medical use in treatment in the United States under federal law and regulations, and have a lack of accepted safety for use under medical supervision.

Federal Law

As has been stated, federal law classifies and regulates marijuana as a Schedule I substance of abuse under the Controlled Substances Act. (10, 11) In fact, a federal court judge recently ruled that marijuana was properly placed in Schedule I. Despite these facts, the current federal government has chosen not to enforce the Drug Substances Act for marijuana and not to prosecute users in states that have chosen to ignore the Act's provisions. The ethical and legal implications of marijuana use have resulted in complicated dilemmas. Sales of marijuana are taxed at the state levels and have exceeded 20%. In one month in 2014, Colorado collected over $2 million in tax revenue. Washington's marijuana tax is approximately 30-40%. The "legalization" of marijuana seems very similar to the "speed cameras" cash cow. The states justify the collection of millions of dollars from the use of speed cameras for the safety of its citizens, while the collection of millions of dollars from marijuana taxes will be used also to benefit society, for example, to fund schools and to remediate the problems that marijuana causes.

Consequences of Marijuana Use

Based on our professional experience and knowledge (the primary author has been a pharmacist for almost 50 years), we summarize the following as consequences of marijuana use, not only for pregnant women, but for all users of this drug substance: (12-16)

- Exposure to marijuana smoke is potentially hazardous and is at least as toxic as cigarette smoke.
- Current evidence indicates that marijuana use during both pregnancy and lactation may adversely affect neurodevelopment, especially critical brain growth after birth and during adolescent maturation.
- Marijuana impacts neuropsychiatric, behavioral, and executive functioning, which may affect future adult productivity and lifetime outcomes (delinquency, depression, and substance abuse).
- Laws passed in States that make recreational use of marijuana legal, render toxicology interpretation complex (is mother using recreational and / or medical marijuana "legally" or illicitly and thus exposing her breastfed baby to "legal" or illicit marijuana?).
- From both philosophical and scientific viewpoints, marijuana should be contraindicated during pregnancy and breastfeeding, as it is hazardous, not only to the unborn baby and nursling, but to the mother as well.
- One aspect of the pro and con sides of the medical and / or legal questions on marijuana use that everyone should agree on is that there is a great need for more empirical data based on scientific studies and labeling that all current prescription and over-the counter (OTC) drugs must undergo before legal and medical use by patients; thus, its use is controversial at best.

The reader may infer that the authors are biased in their conclusions on the use of marijuana while pregnant or breastfeeding. After all, it appears some experts believe the data is not conclusive on increased risks to pregnant women and unborn children. There are those in the breastfeeding community that believe the benefits of breastfeeding and of marijuana use outweigh the risks of artificial formula and marijuana use (see Interview above). So where does the truth about marijuana really lie? To give the reader what the authors believe to be readily available public access, fair, peer-reviewed, accurate, and independent data on marijuana and its use, information from Drugs.Com is provided in Appendix 2. (1) It is highly recommended that readers thoroughly read Appendix 2 and then make their own fair, accurate, and independent determination of just where the truth lies.

Counseling Pregnant Women

How do we counsel pregnant mothers who are using or desire to use marijuana (medically, legally, and / or illicitly)? First of all, there is always the need and recommendation for more studies to research the possible effects of marijuana on the unborn, but that does not help us in the present. Let us once again reiterate: Apparent negative health results during pregnancy include babies born with attention problems, memory problems, and problem solving issues. Several studies have shown no increased risk for miscarriage rates, types of presentation at birth, Apgar status, neonatal complications, or major physical abnormalities, although heavy users reported true ocular hypertelorism (increased distance between the eyes) and severe epicanthus (a vertical fold of skin on either side of the nose). The reality is that the small number of studies has failed to identify major birth defects, while at the same time, it is a fact that marijuana does cross the placental barrier. The ideal plan would be for pregnant women not to use marijuana, but reality usually prevails. There are no statutes that specifically criminalize drug use during pregnancy, but women have been prosecuted under other statutes related to the act of "delivering" drugs to minors. The best case would be to inform the mother of all of these potential scenarios if she wishes to continue to use marijuana during her pregnancy.

Counseling Breastfeeding Women

How do we counsel breastfeeding mothers who are using or desire to use marijuana (medically, legally, and / or illicitly)? We can use the following considerations for honest, compassionate, and informative care of the breastfeeding mother and her child:

- The long-term effects of marijuana on breastfed infants are not entirely known.

- Experts advise that mothers who use marijuana must stop breastfeeding or ask for medical assistance to stop its use, in order for the mother to provide her baby with all the benefits of human milk.

- Some mothers who smoke marijuana away from the baby do not realize the THC from the marijuana is concentrated in breast milk and is absorbed by the nursing babies.

- When mothers are informed of that fact, they may be more willing to give up marijuana for the benefit of their babies.

Recommendations

Based on these considerations, what recommendations can we offer to the mother and her family? In a personal communication with Dr. Thomas Hale on October 19, 2015, Dr. Hale made these suggestions:

- Stop using marijuana while breastfeeding as it could potentially be hazardous. (Primary author's note: no matter what the mother's personal social or health situation for using marijuana, the mother risks losing her child to social services, which would be hazardous to the mother's intimate relationship with her baby through breastfeeding.)

- If the mother is drug screen positive during delivery, stop using marijuana and begin to breastfeed postnatally. (Primary author's note: the amount of marijuana transmitted through colostrum in the days after birth would be minimal because of the small volume of colostrum that the newborn receives as compared to mature milk volume later.)

- The pediatrician should do a drug screen on the infant at one month to determine if the mother has been compliant. (Primary author's note: cannabinoids after a single use can be detected from two to eight days, while chronic use can be detected from five to 30 days. Time for detection increases with increased body fat.)

- The risks in a drug-screen positive mother who used marijuana previously is minimal to the newborn, as long as the mother discontinues its use following delivery.

Summary

In summary, women who use marijuana while pregnant and during breastfeeding should be advised on what is currently known and not known concerning the potential adverse effects on especially fetal growth and development and encouraged to stop using or decrease their use. Long-term follow-up of exposed children is crucial. Potential neurocognitive and behavioral problems may benefit from early recognition and intervention.

Chapter 7: Schedule II, III, IV, V, and Non-Schedule Drugs

Frank J. Nice

One case I often describe in my presentations, related to drug use, was a mom who spoke to a Public Health Nurse (PHN) and admitted she had used Meth.

She was referred to me by an IBCLC in the Maternal and Child Health Program, where I educated nurses and other staff about breastfeeding. We talked about her past use, she did not plan to use after delivery as she wanted to breastfeed. Even so, I discussed with her the risks to her baby of using this drug. We talked about what she would do if she DID use, primarily addressing who would care for her baby and what her baby could have instead of her breast milk. We talked about pumping and storing her milk as a backup or having some formula, and also that if she was breastfeeding and used meth, she would need to "pump and dump" to avoid engorgement, plugged ducts, or mastitis, but this milk would not be safe for her baby.

Months later I got a call from her on a Monday morning. She had used on Friday, her baby was with her mother, and she was pumping and dumping, but wanted to know when she could go back to breastfeeding. This was before these drugs were in *Medications and Mothers' Milk*, so I called Dr. Hale and actually heard from him…..5 days!

I called her back, she said she would.

The PHN later reported to me that this was the only set-back. After that, she continued to breastfeed and stayed clean and sober.

I use this as an example of not "watering down" information – and at the same time the importance of being open and accepting, so moms will call and get information.

(Name withheld by request; used with permission)

Introduction

Drug abuse is defined as the habitual taking of addictive or illegal drugs. (1) Illegal drugs are fairly easy to define (although the current use of marijuana strains the definition). Defining just what drugs are addictive is not as easy. Addiction is a state characterized by compulsive engagement in rewarding stimuli, despite adverse consequences. Using this definition of addiction can include legal drugs, prescription drugs, controlled substance drugs, non-controlled substance drugs, OTCs, herbals, supplements, and recreational substances, among others. Controlled substances pose the most risk to all users, and especially to pregnant and breastfeeding women. This is so not only for reasons already covered, but also because they are among the most common class of drugs to be most commonly abused. The three classes of prescription drugs that are most commonly abused are:

> 1. Opioids, which are most often prescribed to treat pain;
> 2. Central nervous system (CNS) depressants, which are used to treat anxiety and sleep disorders; and
> 3. Stimulants, which are prescribed to treat the sleep disorder narcolepsy and attention-deficit hyperactivity disorder (ADHD).

Schedule II, III, IV, V, and Non-Schedule Drugs

Drug and substances classes (and specific drugs / substances in each class) to be reviewed in this chapter include the following controlled and noncontrolled prescription and OTC medication substances: alcohol, amphetamines, anabolic steroids, analgesics, androgens, anesthetics, antitussives, barbiturates, benzodiazepines, cannabinoids, anti-anxiety carbamates, general anesthetics, methylxanthines, nicotine, nonbarbiturate hypnotics, opioids, pituitary hormones, skeletal muscle relaxants, and stimulants. (2-4)

Alcohol (Ethanol): (5-8) People drink alcohol for many reasons: socializing, celebrating, relaxing, or enhancing a good meal. Alcohol can have a strong effect on people, those who drink and those who are around those who drink. The effect of alcohol depends on many factors: how much you drink, how often you drink, your age, your sex, your ethnicity, your health status, and your family history. Many of those who abuse drug substances are multi-drug users. Alcohol is often one of those substances. When one reads the reviews of drug substances that are abused, one will notice that there are additional negative health effects in combination with alcohol use. Current alcohol use among pregnant women is 8.5%, binge drinking is 2.7%, and heavy drinking is 0.3%. There are no hard statistics on breastfeeding women who use illicit drugs, but it is believed that a similar percentage of women who use alcohol during pregnancy will also use illicit drugs while breastfeeding.

Fetal Alcohol Effects (FAE), which include numerous child developmental and behavioral effects, can result from one to two drinks per day and occasional binge drinking. Fetal Alcohol Syndrome (FAS) can result from heavy drinking of four to six drinks per day. FAS encompasses CNS disorders, including mental retardation, low birth weight, high mortality rate, and structural abnormalities, which include facial dysmorphogenesis, cardiac septal defects, joint abnormalities, hearing issues, urinary problems, eye abnormalities, immune system deficiencies, and skeletal problems. There is no evidence that even several episodes of drinking during the early weeks of pregnancy cause fetal effects. If taken on rare occasions, alcohol should be consumed with food. One to two drinks per day has been linked with prematurity, increased risk of miscarriage, low birth weight, and labor and delivery complications. Therefore, it appears that there is no "safe" amount to consume, and that it is best to just abstain.

Fetal Alcohol Structural Abnormalities

Figure 7.1 FAS Facial Characteristics

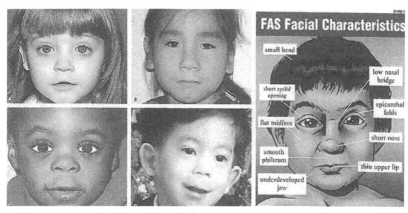

Photo courtesy of University of Maryland Eastern Shore School of Pharmacy

The guidelines for "safe" use during breastfeeding are different from those for pregnancy:

- Alcohol rapidly exchanges between plasma and breast milk.
- One study has shown that mothers' alcohol intake resulted in a 23% reduction in the amount of milk ingested by babies, which may be due to the taste of alcohol in the breast milk.
- Prolactin production may be inhibited by alcohol but this is definitely not known.
- Maternal alcohol blood levels have to reach 300 mg% (mg% is used to designate concentration of alcohol in blood) before significant side effects affect the baby.

- Breastfeeding can be resumed after moderate alcohol use as soon as the mother feels normal.
- Recommend interrupting breastfeeding for two (2) hours per drink or until the mother is sober.
- Excessive chronic drinking can cause mild sedation to deep sleep and hypoprothrombinemic bleeding in breastfed children.
- Intoxicated mothers should not breastfeed; chronic alcoholics should not breastfeed.
- Because the rational use of alcohol is possible during breastfeeding, the use of Alcohol Breast Milk Tests is a waste of money, time, and effort.

Alcohol Dependency Agent: disulfiram (see Chapter 9)

Amphetamines (including amphetamine-related): (5) Amphetamine, benzphetamine, dextroamphetamine, dextroamphetamine / amphetamine (combination), lisdexamfetamine dimesylate, methamphetamine (9), methylphenidate, phendimetrazine, and propylhexedrine (OTC)

Amphetamines are medications that increase alertness, attention, energy, blood pressure, heart rate, and breathing rate. Legal prescription uses for amphetamines include attention-deficit / hyperactivity disorder (ADHD), cataplexy / narcolepsy, narcolepsy, obesity, simple obesity, and moderate to severe binge eating. Note: Methamphetamine can be an extremely addictive stimulant drug. Note: Propylhexedrine is used for nasal congestion, but can be abused to produce stimulation and to increase energy effects.

Health effects include increased wakefulness and physical activity; increased alertness, attention, and energy; decreased appetite; increased breathing, heart rate, blood pressure, and dangerously high temperature; irregular heartbeat; heart problems; heart failure; seizures; narrowed blood vessels; increased blood sugar; opened-up breathing passages; anxiety; anger; confusion; insomnia; mood problems; violent behavior; paranoia; psychoses; hallucinations; delusions; weight loss; severe dental problems (methamphetamine "meth mouth"); and intense itching leading to skin sores from scratching, in addition to risk of HIV, hepatitis, and other infectious diseases from shared needles. Additional health issues in pregnancy include premature delivery, separation of the placenta from the uterus, low birth rate, lethargy, and heart and brain problems, in addition to the shared needles complications. In combination with alcohol, amphetamines can mask the depressant action of alcohol, increase the risk of alcohol overdose, and may increase blood pressure and jitters. Levels of amphetamines in breast milk have been difficult to obtain due to their large volume of distribution in the mothers' bodies. Prescription use of amphetamines seems appropriate for mothers who are breastfeeding. The possibility of breastfed infant irritability and poor sleep patterns exists for prescription use of amphetamines and should be monitored. Abuse of amphetamines by breastfeeding mothers can result in hypertension, palpitations, over-stimulation, motor incoordination, tremor, and restlessness in breastfed babies. Smoked methamphetamine produces similar breast milk concentrations as intravenous methamphetamine use. Breastfeeding can be initiated safely when urine methamphetamine screens are negative for 24 hours. Treatment and screening are necessary for continued promotion of breastfeeding.

Anabolic Steroids: (10) nandrolone, oxandrolone, oxymetholone, and stanozolol

Anabolic steroids are used to treat steroid hormone deficiency, weight gain, antithrombin III deficiency, cryofibrinogenemia, hereditary angioedema, lichen sclerosus et atrophicus, lipodermatosclerosis, Protein C deficiency disease, Raynaud's phenomenon, rheumatoid arthritis, thrombosis, urticaria, anemia of chronic renal failure, acquired aplastic anemia, antineoplastic adverse reaction (myelosuppression), Fanconi's anemia, and pure red cell aplasia. Despite all these exotic conditions that anabolic steroids are used to treat, others abuse these drug substances to enhance athletic and sexual performance and physical appearance. Anabolic steroid use, particularly during the first trimester of pregnancy, may cause virilization of the external genitalia of the female fetus. There are no apparent statistics on steroid abuse in pregnant or breastfeeding women, but as with all abuse substances, their use cannot be ruled out. Long-term steroid use can affect brain pathways and chemicals and affect mood and behavior. Abuse may lead to aggression and psychiatric problems, extreme mood swings, including manic-like symptoms and anger, paranoid jealousy, extreme irritability, delusions, and impaired judgment. In females, health effects include growth of facial hair, male-pattern baldness, changes in or cessation of the menstrual cycle, enlargement of the clitoris, and deepened voice. Those who inject steroids also incur the risk of contracting and transmitting HIV/AIDS or hepatitis. Anabolic steroid use in pregnant and breastfeeding women is definitively contraindicated. Anabolic steroids use may prohibit prolactin production, but not much else has been reported on their abuse and/or abuse during pregnancy. As for pregnancy, anabolic steroids are contraindicated while breastfeeding due to their potential toxic effects on the infant.

Anesthetics: cocaine (topical) (5) and ketamine (11)

There is a case report of a breastfed infant having apnea (suspension of breathing) and seizures after ingesting cocaine applied to the nipple as an anesthetic. Application to other parts of the body, whether breastfeeding or pregnant, results in insignificant plasma levels.

Ketamine is a dissociative (hallucinogens that disrupt or breakdown memory, awareness, identity, or perception) mainly used as an anesthetic in veterinary practice. Adverse health effects include problems with attention, learning, and memory; dreamlike states; hallucinations; sedation; confusion, problems speaking; loss of memory; movement problems leading to immobility; hypertension; ulcers and bladder pain; kidney problems; stomach pain; depression; unconsciousness; and slowed breathing that can lead to death. There is also the risk of HIV, hepatitis, and other infectious diseases from shared needles. In combination with alcohol, there is an increased risk of these ketamine adverse effects. Ketamine use during pregnancy has been associated with newborn depression, increased tone of newborn skeletal muscle, apnea, small size for gestational age, intrauterine growth retardation, hypotonia, and poor reflex responses. Normal ketamine doses result in minimal breastfeeding issues, although the infant should be monitored for sedation, irritability, poor feeding, and weight loss. Ketamine abuse during pregnancy and breastfeeding is possible and has occurred.

Antitussives: camphor (12) (plus nasal decongestant and expectorant) and dextromethorphan (13)

Camphor is a natural product derived from the wood of a tree. Camphor is mostly used medicinally in the form of inhalants and camphorated oil as an antitussive, nasal decongestant and expectorant (helps expel phlegm). At one time the eating of camphor enjoyed some degree of popularity. Today, when it is used, camphor is used as a tincture or powdered camphor is mixed with marijuana and smoked. Ingestion of one gram of camphor will produce a slight stimulating effect, since camphor irritates nerve endings. Users will experience a pleasant, tingly feeling on the skin, some mild restlessness, and a highly excited mental state. Adverse effects include CNS stimulation, convulsions, lethargy, severe nausea, vomiting, hepatotoxicity, and coma. Doses of camphor up to one gram administered to animals have shown no mutations or malformations. Camphor does cross the placental barrier and should be avoided. Used topically and on small areas of the body (not as a substance of abuse), camphor is probably safe for use in breastfeeding mothers.

Dextromethorphan is an antitussive (prevent or relieve a cough) available in OTC and prescription products. It is readily available over the counter in a plethora of products. Using the recommended dose results in few side effects, primarily drowsiness. Recently, illicit use and abuse of dextromethorphan has increased. Recreational users use it to experience a

75

sense of heightened perceptual awareness, altered time perception, complete body dissociation, and visual, auditory, and tactile hallucinations. High doses can cause liver damage, heart attack, stroke, and death, especially when the dextromethorphan is combined with multiple ingredients to also treat other cold and allergy symptoms. The list of other potential adverse effects is prodigious: hot flashes, nausea and dizziness, lack of coordination, panic attack or seizures, impaired judgment and mental performance, numbness, dizziness, sweating, lethargy, hyperactivity, slurred speech, hypertension, nystagmus (rapid eye movement), vomiting, tachycardia, euphoria, paranoia, confusion, disorientation, altered visual disturbances, feelings of floating, movement problems, buildup of excess acid in body fluids, breathing problems, and seizures. In combination with alcohol and other illicit drugs, dextromethorphan procures a synergistic effect. There is little or no data on the placental or mammary transfer of dextromethorphan or on its abuse during pregnancy or breastfeeding. Extrapolating the alcohol abuse statistics for pregnant women, one can assume that there are pregnant and breastfeeding women who abuse dextromethorphan. Dextromethorphan does not appear to have any major teratogenic effects, but the abuse of dextromethorphan has not been studied as a potential for causing teratogenicity. Any breastfed infant whose mother is using dextromethorphan should be monitored for sedation.

Barbiturates: amobarbital, butalbital, butalbital / acetaminophen / caffeine, butalbital / acetaminophen / caffeine / codeine, butalbital / aspirin / caffeine, butalbital /aspirin / caffeine / codeine, methohexital, pentobarbital, phenobarbital, secobarbital, and thiopental

Barbiturates have many medical uses, which include short-term management of insomnia, sedation, premedication for anesthetic procedures, preoperative sedation, headaches, tension-type headaches, muscular headaches, anesthesia, general anesthesia, regional anesthesia, for emergency control of certain acute convulsive episodes (seizures), epilepsy, narcoanalysis, increased intracranial pressure, and complex of tension or muscle contraction. Barbiturates are one class of tranquilizers and depressants (others include benzodiazepines and sleep medications) that slow brain activity, which in turn makes them useful for treating anxiety and sleep problems. When one notes the potential medical uses of barbiturates, one sees many other extended applications. Health effects of barbiturate abuse include drowsiness, slurred speech, poor concentration, confusion, dizziness, movement and memory problems, lowered blood pressure (hypotension), slowed breathing, and many long-term unknown effects. There is also the added risk of HIV, hepatitis, and other infectious disease from shared needles. In combination with alcohol, added risks include further slowing of the heart rate and breathing, which can lead to death. Used during pregnancy, barbiturate withdrawal can cause a serious Neonatal Abstinence Syndrome (NAS) (see Chapter 8) that may even include seizures. Fortunately, barbiturate use during pregnancy is relatively uncommon, and no teratogenic effects have been associated with abuse. Butalbital is one of the most commonly used barbiturates by women, especially for migraine headaches, and some of these women who are heavy users continue its abuse during pregnancy. Using butalbital as an example barbiturate, it apparently transfers into breast milk in limited degrees, although there is no hard data. It should be remembered that butalbital is often combined with acetaminophen, aspirin, caffeine, and/or codeine, which would make abuse of these combinations much more dangerous for a breastfed child. Whether in combination or not, use of these products during breastfeeding warrants monitoring of the infant for sedation, slowed breathing rate, apnea, and pallor.

Benzodiazepines: alprazolam, chlordiazepoxide, clobazam, clonazepam, diazepam, estazolam, halazepam, lorazepam, midazolam, oxazepam, quazepam, and triazolam

Like their older "cousins," the barbiturates, benzodiazepines also have a plethora of medical indications that include anxiety; panic disorder, with or without agoraphobia (sufferer perceives certain environments as dangerous or uncomfortable); alcohol withdrawal syndrome; benzodiazepine withdrawal; skeletal muscle spasm; Lennox-Gastaut Syndrome (adjunct treatment for seizures); seizures; status epilepticus (continuous seizures); insomnia; insomnia due to anxiety or situational stress; premedication for anesthetic procedures; induction of amnesia; preoperative sedation; and sedation for a mechanically ventilated patient. Like the barbiturates, benzodiazepine abuse can cause drowsiness, slurred speech, poor concentration, confusion, dizziness, movement and memory problems, lowered blood pressure (hypotension), slowed breathing, and many long-term unknown effects. There is also the added risk of HIV, hepatitis, and other infectious disease from shared needles. In combination with alcohol, added risks include further slowing of the heart rate and breathing, which can lead to death. During pregnancy, because the fetal exposure of benzodiazepines has been extensively studied, it is known that the risk of abuse of these substances is relatively high. There is an apparent risk of multiple anomalies, including cleft lip, fetal growth restriction, and intrauterine death. Benzodiazepine use during pregnancy is usually associated with other substance abuse, including alcohol and tobacco. One could make the assumption of similar benzodiazepine abuse during breastfeeding. Abrupt discontinuation, though, during pregnancy or breastfeeding, should be avoided due to severe maternal withdrawal symptoms and suicidal ideation.

Breastfed babies of abusers should be especially monitored for sedation, slowed breathing rate, not waking to feed, poor feeding, and poor weight gain.

Cannabinoids: dronabinol and nabilone

Synthetic cannabinoids are cannabinoids structurally related to THC. Two controlled cannabinoid substances, dronabinol and nabilone are currently marketed as prescription drugs. They are basically synthetic substitutes for marijuana. Unlike "medical" and "legal" marijuana, they have undergone all the necessary clinical trials based on research and scientific data for safety and effectiveness. This describes their medical prescription status. Cannabinoids have the same abuse potential as marijuana and similar mechanisms of action and thus adverse health effects, including pregnancy and breastfeeding. In addition, clinical doses used short-term apparently are compatible with breastfeeding, while the long-term use of cannabinoids should be avoided and is not recommended. If used medically, the breastfed infant should be monitored for sedation, changes in sleep pattern, irritability, and weight gain. The reader is referred to Chapter 6 and Appendix 2.

There are misleadingly labeled synthetic cannabinoids that are not prescription drugs marketed as natural, safe, and legal alternatives to marijuana. These include a wide variety of herbal mixtures containing man-made cannabinoid chemicals also related to THC, but often much stronger and more dangerous. These dangers include increased heart rate, vomiting, agitation, confusion, hallucinations, anxiety, paranoia, hypertension, reduced blood supply to the heart, and heart attack. The long-term effects are currently unknown as are the use of these substances in combination with alcohol.

Carbamates (Anti-anxiety): meprobamate (14) and meprobamate / aspirin

Meprobamate is a drug that has been around for a long time. It was one of the original drugs developed for anxiety and was first synthesized in 1950. It still finds use for anxiety, tense feelings, and as an adjunct drug for pain. Physical dependence, psychological dependence, and abuse have occurred. When chronic intoxication from prolonged use occurs, it usually involves ingestion of greater than recommended doses and is manifested by ataxia, slurred speech, and vertigo. Sudden withdrawal of the drug after prolonged and excessive use may precipitate recurrence of pre-existing symptoms, such as anxiety, anorexia, and insomnia, or withdrawal reactions, such as vomiting, ataxia (full loss of bodily movement), tremors, muscle twitching, confusional states, hallucinations, and rarely, convulsive seizures. Such seizures are more likely to occur in persons with central nervous system damage or pre-existent or latent convulsive disorders.

An increased risk of congenital malformations associated with the use meprobamate during the first trimester of pregnancy has been suggested in several studies. Meprobamate passes the placental barrier. It is present both in umbilical cord blood close to maternal plasma levels and in breast milk of lactating mothers at concentrations two to four times that of maternal plasma. Because sedation at these levels is possible in the infant, use of meprobamate should be avoided as safer anti-anxiety agents become available for treatment. Overall, the use of meprobamate should be highly discouraged during pregnancy and breastfeeding at any level of use or abuse.

Laxatives: (15) saline, senna

Because of the higher incidence of constipation during pregnancy and while breastfeeding, women may misuse or abuse laxatives. Another reason for laxative abuse is the condition of bulimia nervosa, which is a serious, potentially life-threatening eating disorder characterized by a cycle of bingeing and compensatory behaviors, such as self-induced vomiting, designed to undo or compensate for the effects of binge eating. One of the consequences of bulimia is chronic irregular bowel movements and constipation as a result of laxative abuse. Bulimia nervosa affects 1-2% of adolescent and young adult women, and approximately 80% of bulimia nervosa patients are female. The main health effects of laxative abuse are electrolyte imbalances that can lead to irregular heartbeat and possibly heart failure and death. Electrolyte imbalance is caused by dehydration and loss of potassium and sodium from the body as a result of laxative purging behaviors. These electrolyte imbalances can have direct effects on the fetus and breastfed baby. Lethargy, confusion, weakness, swelling, seizures, coma lethargy, nausea, vomiting, diarrhea, sweating, abnormal electrical conduction in the heart and potentially life-threatening heart rhythm problems, kidney failure, kidney stones, abdominal pain, depression, muscle spasms, and heart rhythm disturbances, muscles with weakness and cramps, hallucinations, muscle weakness, breathing difficulties and acid-base disturbances can result from electrolyte imbalances. Appropriate use of most laxatives is compatible with pregnancy and breastfeeding.

Methylxanthine: caffeine

Caffeine use during pregnancy is probably safe when used in moderate amounts. Data suggest no known association between caffeine use and poor fetal outcomes. Maternal use of more than 500 mg/day may have some association with fetal cardiac arrhythmias as compared to 250 mg per day.

Even though clearance of caffeine in infants is markedly reduced, amounts ingested by breastfeeding children are small if the mother uses reasonable amounts of coffee, tea, or colas (one to two cups per day). Mothers of newborns, and in particular of premature newborns whose enzyme metabolism is still immature, should avoid caffeine. Possible caffeine induced effects to monitor in infants are agitation, irritability, poor sleeping patterns, rapid heartbeat, and tremors. Mothers who are taking theophylline (for asthma) should use caution due to the synergistic effects of theophylline with caffeine.

The following caffeine usage guide for users is offered for pregnant and breastfeeding women:

Table 7.1 Caffeine Usage Guide

SUBSTANCE	CAFFEINE CONTENT (mg)
Pure Caffeine	
Caffeine Powder (1/16 teaspoon)	200
Liquid Caffeine (0.08 oz)	41.5
Coffee (5 oz cup)	
Drip method	110-150
Percolated	64-124
Instant	40-108
Decaffeinated	2-5
Instant Decaffeinated	2
Tea (5 oz cup)	
1 minute brew	9-33
3 minute brew	20-46
5 minute brew	20-50
Instant tea	12-28
Iced tea (12 oz cup)	22-36
Soft Drink/Soda (12 oz serving)	
Jolt	72.0
Sugar-Free Mr Pibb	58.8

Mountain Dew	54.0
Mountain Zevia	55.0
Mello Yello	52.8
Tab	46.8
Coca-Cola	45.6
Coca-Cola Life	27.0
Coke	45.6
Coca Cola Zero	36.0
Diet Coke	45.6
Shasta Cola	44.4
Shasta Cherry Cola	44.4
Shasta Diet Cola	44.4
Shasta Diet Cherry Cola	44.4
Surge	52.5
Mr Pibb	40.8
Pibb Xtra	40.8
Dr Pepper	39.6
Big Red	38.4
Sugar-Free Dr Pepper	39.6
Pepsi-Cola	38.4
Aspen	36.0
Diet Pepsi	36.0
Pepsi Light	36.0
Pepsi MAX	69.0
Pepsi True	38.4
RC Cola	36.0
Diet Rite	36.0
Kick	31.2
Canada Dry Jamaica Cola	30.0

Canada Dry Diet Cola	1.2
Barq's Root Beer	23.0
Energy Drinks	
Bang Energy Drink (16 oz)	367
Redline Energy Drink (8 oz)	316
Rockstar (16 oz)	160
Rockstar Citrus Punched (16 oz)	240
5-Hour Energy (1.9 oz)	208
Full Throttle (16 oz)	200
Frava Caffeinated Juice (16 oz)	200
Monster Energy (16 oz)	160
Venom Energy Drink (16 oz)	160
NOS Energy Drink (16 oz)	160
AMP Energy Boost Original (16 oz)	142
NoDoz Energy Shots (1.89 oz)	115
Mountain Dew Kick Start (16 oz)	92
Avitae Caffenated Water (16.9 oz)	90
Red Bull (8.4 oz)	80
V8 V-Fusion+Energy (8 oz)	80
Ocean Spray Cran-Energy (20 oz)	55
Glaceau Vitaminwater Energy (20 oz)	50
Starbucks Refreshers (12 oz)	50
MIO Energy (1 squirt/1/2 tsp)	60
Crystal Light Energy (1/2 packet)	60
Over-the-Counter (OTC'S)	
Zantrex-3-Weight Loss (2 capsules)	300
NoDoz (1 caplet)	200
Vivarin (2 tablets)	200
Excedrin Migraine (2 yablets)	130

Midol Complete (2 caplets)	120
Bayer Back & Body (2 caplets)	65
Anacin (2 tablets)	64

Nicotine: Tobacco (5)

Tobacco, whose main active ingredient is nicotine, is a plant grown for its leaves, which are then dried and fermented before use. There are an additional 4,000 chemicals, including 43 known carcinogens, produced during smoking. Nicotine readily crosses the placenta resulting in higher fetal levels than maternal levels. Tobacco use during pregnancy is approximately 13% to 15%. The rate is probably very similar for breastfeeding women. Nicotine also passes into breast milk, and smoking during the postpartum period causes a significant health risk for both the mother and her child. Adverse health effects of tobacco usage include increased blood pressure; increased breathing rate; increased heart rate; a greatly increased risk of cancer, especially lung cancer when smoked and oral cancer when chewed; chronic bronchitis; heart disease; leukemia; cataracts; and pneumonia. Use during pregnancy can result in miscarriage, malnutrition, low birth weight, fetal hypoxia-ischemia, premature delivery, stillbirth, and learning and behavior problems. The effects of concomitant alcohol use are presently unknown. In utero exposure to smoking during pregnancy may increase the risk of diabetes and obesity resulting in lifelong metabolic disorders. The use of nicotine patches to help stop smoking postpartum is compatible with breastfeeding (as long as the mother does not continue to smoke while on the patch) as no untoward effects have been observed with breastfeeding babies in a nicotine patch study.

Non-Barbiturate Hypnotics: chloral hydrate, eszopiclone, ramelteon, zaleplon, and zolpidem

Similar to barbiturates in actions and adverse reactions and health effects, these "sleep medications" slow brain activity, which makes them useful for treating (and in the case of chloral hydrate, also for sedating patients) sleep disorders. Short-term effects include drowsiness (including the next day after taking at bedtime), slurred speech, poor concentration, confusion, dizziness, movement and memory problems, hypotension, and slowed breathing, while long-term effects are unknown. These sleep medications are sometimes abused as "date rape" drugs. Use in combination with alcohol can lead to further slowing of the heart rate and breathing, which can lead to death. Chloral hydrate was first synthesized in 1832, while the other agents in this

83

category are fairly new. There is inadequate information on the use of these drugs during pregnancy and breastfeeding. It is well known that one of the main risks of taking chloral hydrate is addiction. Once addicted, attempts to stop can lead to a difficult withdrawal syndrome, which is so dangerous that most people need to enter a medical facility. Other characteristics of addiction include drug cravings, building a tolerance to chloral hydrate, and psychological dependency on the drug. As for the other agents, abuse leads to benzodiazepine-like results.

It is recommended that these drugs only be used in pregnancy if the benefits outweigh the risks. This advice is not very helpful for legal prescription use, but it does portend a conclusion that abuse during pregnancy definitely poses risks to the fetus. As for breastfeeding, prescription chloral hydrate is apparently compatible, but the infant needs to be monitored for sedation, slowed breathing rate, not waking to feed, poor feeding, and weight gain. Similar monitoring of the infant is also needed for the other agents in this drug category. These potential breastfed-baby effects would certainly be exacerbated by maternal abuse of the drug substances.

Opioids: (5) belladonna / opium, carisoprodol / aspirin / codeine, chlorpheniramine polistirex / codeine, codeine, codeine / acetaminophen, codeine / aspirin, codeine phosphate / guaifenesin, difenoxin hydrochloride / atropine, dihydrocodeine, dihydrocodeine / aspirin / caffeine, diluted tincture of opium (paregoric), diphenoxylate hydrochloride / atropine, fentanyl, hydrocodone, hydrocodone bitartrate / hydrocodone methylbromide, hydrocodone bitartrate / acetaminophen, hydrocodone bitartrate / chlorpheniramine, hydrocodone bitartrate / guaifenesin, hydrocodone bitartrate / ibuprofen, hydrocodone bitartrate / pseudoephedrine, hydrocodone / chlorpheniramine / pseudoephedrine, hydrocodone polistirex / chlorpheniramine, hydromorphone, levophanol, meperidine, methadone (see Chapter 9), morphine, morphine sulfate / naltrexone, nalbuphine, oxycodone, oxycodone / acetaminophen, oxycodone/aspirin, oxycodone hydrochloride / naloxone hydrochloride, oxycodone / ibuprofen, oxymorphone, promethazine hydrochloride / codeine, promethazine / phenylephrine / codeine, remifentanil, sufentanil, tapentadol, tramadol, and tramadol hydrochloride / acetaminophen.

Opioids have wide use (the United States population used more narcotic drugs than the rest of the worlds' patients combined) for acute pain, moderate to severe acute pain, severe chronic pain, chronic pain, moderate to moderately severe pain, moderate to severe pain, moderate to severe ureteric pain, intractable pain, postoperative pain, dental pain, musculoskeletal pain, obstetric pain, analgesia in labor, epidural analgesia, pain not responsive to nonnarcotic analgesics, breakthrough cancer pain, in patients requiring a daily around-the-clock analgesic, in patients requiring long-term daily continuous opioid analgesia, diarrhea, in opioid tolerant patients, anesthesia, general anesthesia, premedication for procedures, premedication for anesthetic procedures, monitored anesthesia care sedation, cough, cough associated with upper respiratory allergies or a common cold, cough due to minor throat and bronchial irritation, nasal congestion associated with the common cold, nasal congestion associated with upper respiratory allergies, anxiety due to dyspnea associated with pulmonary edema caused by acute left ventricular dysfunction, diabetic peripheral neuropathy, heart failure, and pulmonary emphysema.

The health effects of opioid use are drowsiness, nausea, constipation, euphoria, confusion, slowed breathing, and death. In addition, there is the risk of HIV, hepatitis, and other infectious diseases from shared needles. In combination with alcohol use, there are additional risks of dangerous slowing of the heart rate and breathing leading to coma or death. Most of the information on the effects of opioid use during pregnancy comes from studies on heroin and methadone use. The reported prevalence of opioid use ranges from 1% to 21% (this percentage reflects at-risk populations). Use during pregnancy can result in miscarriage, low birth rate, and Neonatal Abstinence Syndrome (NAS) (see Chapter 8). Most narcotics at appropriate doses, if needed for pain control, can be taken while breastfeeding, but breastfed infants must be closely monitored mainly for sedation, slowed breathing rate, pallor, constipation, and appropriate weight gain. The case of codeine presents another issue: rapid maternal metabolism. The following case report is presented as an example of maternal codeine rapid metabolism to morphine:

> A 13-day old breastfed infant died from morphine overdose when the mother took codeine to treat episiotomy pain. After the death, a genetic test showed the mother to be a rapid metabolizer of codeine. The chance of being a rapid metabolizer ranges from less than 1 per 100 to 28 per 100 people. Only a genetic test can tell if a person is affected, but there is only limited information about using this test for codeine metabolism to morphine. In most cases, codeine is, and continues to be, appropriate treatment for pain while breastfeeding. It should be used at the lowest dose for the shortest period of time. The mother in this case noted excess drowsiness in herself, so the physician lowered the dose, but the drowsiness continued. The mother continued to take the codeine for an extended time. During this time, her baby also

began to experience similar signs because of the high level of morphine in the breast milk. After 13 days, the baby experienced depression and died. It seems apparent that the mother was not counseled properly on the potential adverse effects of codeine (rapid metabolizers or not) on her breastfed child. A mother should never have a breastfed baby in respiratory depression before realizing the medication she is taking has led to the outcome.

Opioid Partial Agonists /Antagonists: buprenorphine (see Chapter 9), buprenorphine / naloxone (see Chapter 9), butorphanol, naloxone (see Chapter 9), naltrexone (see Chapter 9), pentazocine, and pentazocine hydrochloride / naloxone hydrochloride

Partial agonists activate the opioid receptors in the brain, but to a much lesser degree than full or pure agonists (for example, heroin, oxycodone, methadone, hydrocodone, morphine, opium and others). Buprenorphine also acts as an antagonist, meaning it blocks other opioids, while allowing for some opioid effect of its own to suppress withdrawal symptoms and cravings. Agonist drugs block opioids by attaching to the opioid receptors without activating them. Antagonists cause no opioid effect and completely block full agonist opioids. Examples are naltrexone and naloxone. Naloxone is sometimes used to reverse a heroin overdose. This will be further clarified in Chapter 9. This class of opioids can also be used to treat moderate to severe pain, severe chronic pain, labor pain, and for anesthesia. These drugs have a lower abuse potential than the pure agonist opioid analgesics, such as morphine. However, all have been subject to abuse and misuse, and the information presented for opioids are applicable when this group of drugs is abused. As for breastfeeding, data is limited for this class of drugs, but when conducting a comprehensive benefits / risks analysis of the benefits of opioid partial agonists / antagonists plus the benefits of breastfeeding, it is apparent that the benefits outweigh the risks of the drugs and the risks of artificial formula.

Pituitary Hormone: somatrem / somatropin (human growth hormone) (16)

Human growth hormone is used for the treatment of growth hormone deficiency, decreased body growth (Prader-Willi syndrome), short stature disorder (Noonan syndrome), renal function impairment with growth failure, and small-for-gestational-age baby with no catch-up by age two to four years. Human growth hormone is used illicitly to increase athletic performance and for its supposed anti-aging properties. Health risks include acromegaly (abnormal bone growth, enlarged lips, enlarged nose, thickening and widening of forehead and jaw, overbite, separation of teeth, joint swelling and pain, arthritis, excess hair growth, weight gain, enlarged hands and feet, thickened skin, heart disease, and diabetes), acquired Creutzfeldt-Jakob disease (brain disease similar to "mad cow"), and breast enlargement and tumors. Other health risks include hypertension, acne, pancreatitis, leukemia, high blood sugar, carpal tunnel syndrome, high cholesterol and triglycerides, and increased sweating. Human growth hormone has been used to enhance the chances of getting pregnant. The use of human growth hormone is not advised for pregnant or breastfeeding women as can be seen by the extended list of negative health effects of abuse. Regular medically acceptable use during breastfeeding is possible since human growth hormone is a peptide of 191 amino acids with a huge molecular mass of 124,124 Daltons, which would make transfer into breast milk very unlikely. If used, the breastfed infant should be monitored for hypothyroidism and hypoglycemia.

Sedative / Hypnotic: propofol

Propofol is used for general anesthesia and sedation for mechanically ventilated patients, especially in the intensive care unit. As can be seen by the highly publicized use of propofol by a well known and now deceased American singer, songwriter, record producer, dancer, and actor, abuse is very possible. It is also possible for withdrawal symptoms to occur when propofol has been consumed for as short as one to two weeks. Withdrawal symptoms include unpleasant feelings, sweating, nausea, fatigue, insomnia, irritability, stomach cramps, panic attacks, vomiting, tremors, and seizures. Just a "little too much" can result in death. Propofol in prescription doses can be used safely during pregnancy and breastfeeding. Propofol crosses the placental barrier. Thus, it seems appropriate to extrapolate the just a "little too much" results in death for abusers could be possible for the unborn child of a maternal abuser. The breastfed infant should be monitored for sedation, slowed breathing rate, not waking to feed, and poor feeding.

Skeletal Muscle Relaxants: baclofen, carisoprodol (17), chlorzoxazone, cyclobenzaprine (18), metaxalone, methocarbamol, and orphenadrine

Skeletal muscle relaxants are used extensively for skeletal muscle pain, skeletal muscle spasm, disorders of the musculoskeletal system, spasticity, and spasm due to tetanus. Adverse effects include sedation and drowsiness most commonly. These powerful drugs also can cause heart failure and paralysis; confusion and lethargy; fainting; abdominal pain; nausea and vomiting; seizures; headaches; irritability and nervousness; and anticholinergic effects that include dry mouth, constipation, and blurred vision. Carisoprodol (see meprobamate, which is the metabolite of carisoprodol and is also a controlled substance) is currently the only controlled skeletal muscle relaxant substance. Its abuse has increased dramatically in recent years. Abuse effects are similar to those of meprobamate. Carisoprodol withdrawal syndrome exists and includes anxiety, tremors, muscle twitching, insomnia, hallucinations, and bizarre behavior. All of the other skeletal muscle relaxants have the same abuse potential. There is potential for an increased risk of abuse among individuals suffering from depression or mental illness who may be at risk for contemplating or attempting to take their life. As with any substance, abuse is more common among individuals who have a reason to self-medicate, which the use of most skeletal muscle relaxants allow. When muscle spasms are accompanied by acute and chronic pain, these drugs dull the nerve impulses in the human body. The resulting numb and relaxed feelings are very appealing to legitimate users, as well as drug abusers. Currently, the FDA states that no adequate or controlled studies exist in humans for the medical use of skeletal muscle relaxants, so it would seem evident that abuse of these drug substances can be potentially toxic to the fetus and breastfed infant. As for breastfeeding and taking the prescription dosage of skeletal muscle relaxants, their use seems to be probably compatible, but the infant must be monitored for drowsiness, dry mouth, tremor, rigidity, and wide pupils (baclofen); sedation, weakness, vomiting, and hiccups (carisoprodol); lethargy, vomiting, dark urine, and jaundice (chlorzoxazone); drowsiness, dry mouth, and vomiting (cyclobenzaprine); sedation, vomiting, and gastrointestinal upset (metaxalone); drowsiness, vomiting, and fever (methocarbamol); and agitation, dizziness, tremor, dry mouth, and vomiting (orphenadrine).

Chapter 8: Neonatal Abstinence Syndrome (NAS)

Cheryl A. Harrow

Brianna's Story - Neonatal Abstinence Syndrome (NAS)

At the time of delivery, Brianna was taking 2 mg of Dilaudid twice a day, and she was given this amount during her hospital stay, as well as Vicodin, in the days after the birth.

Baby's withdrawal symptoms were measured during a 24-hour window to determine whether he would go home or have a two-week NICU stay, with a weaning dose of morphine. She thinks it was a 0-3 Scale. If he sneezed more than three times in a row, he got one point. She could not really remember the scoring system, but she thinks they took his heart rate as well. She never got a record of what his scores were. She mentioned that she knew they measured sneezing and that they routinely took his vitals. Baby never experienced the worst withdrawal symptoms, such as seizures, though he did have significant twitching at one point. After 24 hours of him scoring fine, they stayed an extra day for jaundice, and then took him home.

"If I was nursing, he was fine; he wasn't sneezing, he kind of would twitch a little bit...; there was really only a 24 hour period where it was touch and go...the doctors were saying that if he does not get his scoring below a certain level, we will have to start him on morphine."

During her pregnancy, Brianna stated that her mantra to her baby was "practice your sucking, practicing your sucking," because she "knew" that comfort nursing would help to get him through the withdrawal.

Brianna felt that in addition to the comfort of breastfeeding, the small amount of narcotics that were present in her breast milk helped to ease baby's withdrawal symptoms. *"I could tell that he was more comfortable after I got my dose.... It was around 6:30 pm that I got my dose, and if I was nursing around 8 pm, I could tell that he was calm. I think that I was the only one who could tell, but he was just more comfortable."*

"It wasn't until we pulled into our driveway, and my mom was there to greet us, that I was assured that we would be able to take this baby home."

(Continued in Chapter 10)

Introduction

Opium has been used since its discovery to treat headaches, pain, heart attacks, vomiting, diarrhea, and surgery, as well as childbirth and female problems (1, 2). For centuries women of childbearing age have become opiate dependent and delivered infants that experience symptoms of withdrawal. In Kandall's (1) review of the literature, he noted Marshall's (3) estimation of the "sales popularity of Mrs. Winslow's Soothing Syrup" (p. 11), and Pettey's (4) description of the clinical signs of "congenital morphinism," the relationship of the clinical signs in the newborn infant to the maternal narcotic amount, and a regimen for the treatment of the infant (p. 42).

In the last decade, increasing numbers of childbearing women are opiate dependent, on maintenance therapy following opiate use, using illicit drugs, and/or abusing licit drugs. This has led to a growing number of newborns with symptoms of drug withdrawal following intrauterine drug exposure, called Neonatal Abstinence Syndrome (NAS) (5, 6).

A comprehensive program can provide on-going support for drug-dependent pregnant women and their infants (7, 8). A comprehensive program begins with entry into prenatal care and stabilization of maternal drug use as well as medical evaluation and treatment, and psychiatric services if needed. Counseling for drug use and support should begin prenatally and continue through the postpartum period. Delivery and care of the mother and her infant after birth should be in an inpatient setting that encourages mothers and infants to remain together, especially if the infant requires pharmacologic treatment, and encourages breastfeeding when feasible. Social services should be available to assess for maternal possession of infant supplies and other social needs of support during hospitalization and after discharge. Identification of a pediatric care provider and a planned first visit should occur prior to discharge, as well as appointments for other needed services. This type of comprehensive care program provides an ideal setting for collection of maternal and fetal/neonatal data to aid future research with the goal of improving outcomes for mothers and infants. In the absence of a comprehensive program, the prenatal and obstetric care providers as well as the pediatrician have the responsibility to report any information mandated by law to social services for further investigation.

World Health Organization (WHO)

The World Health Organization (WHO) recognized a lack of global guidelines with evidence-based recommendations for the identification and management of substance use and substance use disorders during pregnancy, especially in low and middle income countries. The WHO developed guidelines based on the evidence available, for health care providers to manage pregnant women and new mothers, actively using substances, or with substance use disorder, to achieve healthy outcomes for themselves and their children (9). The WHO guidelines focus on screening and brief intervention, psychosocial interventions, detoxification, dependence management, infant feeding, and management of infant withdrawal. In addition, the American Congress of Obstetricians and Gynecologists (ACOG), the American Academy of Pediatrics (AAP), and the Academy of Breastfeeding Medicine (ABM), have written recommendations. This chapter is written to be congruent with the WHO, ACOG, AAP, and ABM.

American College of Obstetricians and Gynecologists (ACOG)

The American College of Obstetricians and Gynecologists (ACOG) Committee on Health Care for Underserved Women and the American Society of Addiction Medicine released their Committee Opinion #524 in 2012 (10). ACOG's recommendation is for women to begin a maintenance therapy, such as methadone or buprenorphine, during pregnancy to eliminate use of illicit or prescription opioids. They also recommended adjusting the maintenance medication dose to keep the pregnant woman asymptomatic due to the changes in metabolism during pregnancy.

American Academy of Pediatrics (AAP)

The American Academy of Pediatrics released a revised policy statement in 2001, making methadone compatible with breastfeeding with the elimination of the dose restriction. The policy statement from 1994 had limited the maternal methadone dose compatible with breastfeeding as ≤ 20 mg a day, which originally eliminated the vast majority of women on methadone maintenance from breastfeeding. The AAP also released a revised statement in 2012 with updates on clinical presentation following intrauterine drug exposure, therapeutic options in treating withdrawal, and included evidence based management approaches to weaning hospitalized infants from analgesics and sedatives (6).

Academy of Breastfeeding Medicine (ABM)

The Academy of Breastfeeding Medicine Protocol Committee revised Clinical Protocol #21: Guidelines for Breastfeeding and the Drug-Dependent Woman in 2015 (see Chapter 4) (11). The purpose of the protocol is to provide literature-based guidelines to evaluate and manage the woman with substance use or substance use disorder who desires to breastfeed her newborn. The protocol addresses methadone and buprenorphine, opioids, marijuana, alcohol, and tobacco, along with the recommendations for breastfeeding. Infant NAS scores, need for replacement opiates, and hospital length of stay have been shown to be decreased in the infants whose mothers chose to breastfeed and met the standard recommendations to breastfeed according to The Academy of Breastfeeding Medicine.

What is Neonatal Abstinence Syndrome?

NAS has been described as a constellation of symptoms involving the central nervous system, gastrointestinal system, respiratory system, and autonomic system (12) following intrauterine exposure to opioids such as heroin, methadone, buprenorphine, oxycodone, and other opioid medication use and misuse. NAS symptoms result from neonatal behavioral dysregulation following prenatal exposure to opioids. This neonatal behavioral dysregulation can also be produced by intrauterine exposure to other substances that are not opioids such as alcohol (13, 14), nicotine (15), benzodiazepines (16, 17), psychiatric medications including antidepressants (6, 18), and marijuana (19). Since the dysregulation presents with the same symptoms, more and / or worse symptoms can be seen with the combined usage of opioids and other medications / substances.

NAS is seen as the collective expression of physiological and behavioral signs an infant may experience following intrauterine exposure to opioids and other substances. The presentation of symptoms varies from infant-to-infant and is not completely understood due to its complexity. During pregnancy, the fetus receives a passive supply of opioids and other substances. As the newborn infant continues to metabolize and excrete the remaining maternal drug(s) and their byproduct(s), there is an increase in the number and severity of symptoms (see Table 8.1, Symptoms of NAS). Clinical features vary in their presentation and usually increase in severity over the first two weeks after birth, with some infants having few and less severe symptoms, while others have more symptoms and / or increased severity. As the maternal drug is metabolized by the infant, neurotransmitters are altered resulting in an imbalance between the sympathetic and parasympathetic systems, which regulate the involuntary body activities.

Self-regulation, using the sympathetic and parasympathetic systems, includes the ability to control sleep and wake states, motor tone, sensory processing, and stress. Over time, these neurotransmitters rebalance and symptoms begin to dissipate. The use of non-pharmacologic interventions can assist the infant by decreasing the number and severity of NAS symptoms (20). The addition of an opiate replacement medication may be necessary if, despite use of non-pharmacological interventions, symptoms continue to interfere with the infant's ability to eat, sleep, and grow. Treatment will be addressed later in this chapter.

The increasing incidence of NAS nearly parallels the increasing incidence of prescription and illicit opioid use during pregnancy. The risk of NAS from opioid use increases with the addition of smoking, stimulants, depressants, and the simultaneous use of other prescribed drugs, such as benzodiazepines and psychotropic medications. Medications used for opioid maintenance therapy in pregnancy are known to result in NAS, but are safer for the fetus than illicit drug use.

Drug Substances That Can Result in NAS Symptoms

Commonly used, misused, or abused drugs in pregnancy that can result in NAS include opioid maintenance therapy medications, opioid analgesics, and heroin. These drugs are not listed by potential to cause NAS, and this list is not all inclusive. For many drugs, there is limited research and existing data on the effects of the drugs on the fetus, newborn, and breastfeeding infant due to legal, social, and ethical issues surrounding infants as a vulnerable population.

Buprenorphine

Buprenorphine is a partial μ-opioid agonist and ϰ-antagonist opioid maintenance medication. Buprenorphine is available by prescription from opioid maintenance therapy programs and community physicians who have obtained the required special Drug Enforcement Agency (DEA) registration number. Buprenorphine is the first drug approved by the Food and Drug Administration for the treatment of opioid use disorder in community-based physician offices. Currently, nurse practitioners and physician assistants cannot obtain the required DEA number. The expanded availability of buprenorphine has resulted in more street-available buprenorphine and the increased possibility of use during pregnancy without a treatment program or prescription. In studies comparing infants prenatally exposed to buprenorphine to matched pairs prenatally exposed to methadone, buprenorphine-exposed infants required significantly less morphine for treatment, shorter length of treatment, and shorter hospital stays than infants exposed to methadone (12, 21, 22).

Routine urine toxicology screening panels generally do not include testing for buprenorphine; therefore, further investigation of buprenorphine use may be warranted in the setting of NAS symptoms without maternal report of use of buprenorphine and negative routine toxicology testing. Buprenorphine is usually dosed between 2 mg and 32 mg daily, has a duration of action of 8 to 12 hours at low doses (e.g., 2 mg), and 24 to 72 hours at higher doses (e.g., >16 mg), with a half-life of 24 to 60 hours. Symptoms of NAS after birth begin in the first few days and can escalate in the first week to two weeks. More research is needed to determine which infants exposed to buprenorphine will need pharmacological treatment and why one infant has minimal symptoms of NAS while another has severe symptoms.

The American College of Obstetricians and Gynecologists (ACOG) Committee (Opinion Number 524, 2012) has no limitation on maternal dosage during pregnancy and lactation due to low concentrations in breast milk and poor bioavailability (5, 23). The ACOG Consensus Panel (2012) stated that breastfeeding is compatible with buprenorphine at any dose and women should be informed that the amount of buprenorphine found in breast milk is minimal so there is likely to be minimal effects on the breastfed infant, despite limited empirical data and the package insert advising against breastfeeding (5).

Methadone

Methadone is a full μ-opioid agonist, and is considered the international standard of care for treatment of opiate-dependent pregnant women. Methadone has been used as opioid maintenance therapy since the 1970s and continues to be widely used (24). Methadone is associated with increased prenatal care and better infant outcomes, such as longer gestational age, higher weight, and fewer complications than with continued use of heroin. Intrauterine exposure to methadone can result in NAS, and has not been found to be maternal dose dependent. Cleary et al. (2010) included 29 studies in his systematic review and meta-analysis looking at the relationship between maternal methadone dose and infants needing treatment for withdrawal after birth, and concluded that infant withdrawal symptoms are not directly related to maternal methadone dose (25). The systematic review and meta-analysis did conclude that a greater likelihood and longer duration of infant treatment was associated with the combination of methadone treatment and concurrent use of other drugs (25). Generally, methadone dosing ranges from 20 mg to 200 mg, however, doses exceeding 200 mg daily may be needed. The duration of action after a single dose of methadone is four to eight hours, and after multiple daily doses may be 22 to 48 hours. The half-life for the elimination of methadone is 8 to 59 hours (26); therefore, the exposed infant may experience few symptoms in the first two days, after which more symptoms develop with increasing severity until about two weeks of age.

The American College of Obstetricians and Gynecologists (ACOG) Committee, Opinion Number 524, 2012 (5) and the American Academy of Pediatrics (6) have no limitation on maternal methadone dose during pregnancy and lactation. The maternal and fetal outcomes of methadone use during pregnancy, versus continued heroin use, are far better, such as enrollment in prenatal care, full-term deliveries, and neonatal well-being. The ACOG Consensus Panel stated that breastfeeding is compatible with methadone at any dose, and there is likely to be minimal effects on the breastfed infant because of the low concentrations found in breast milk (5). Past studies have found the amount of methadone in breast milk to be minimal, and current studies using new technology have confirmed earlier findings (27). Breastfed infants benefit from the comfort of the act of breastfeeding, and this comforting helps to lessen the severity of symptoms. This effect may be interpreted as providing methadone through breast milk; however, the concentration of methadone in breast milk has found to be less than one percent up to six percent of the maternal dose and not enough to treat symptoms of withdrawal (23).

Opiates

Multiple opiate medications prescribed during pregnancy, or misused, in addition to heroin use, can result in NAS symptoms after birth (see Table 8.2, Opiate Duration of Action and Half-Life). Onset of NAS after birth is related to multiple factors including duration of action, half-life for elimination, timing of last dose, number of doses per day, and length of time used. Concurrent use of other drugs will also affect the expression of NAS symptoms.

Breastfeeding is contraindicated while using heroin, while using opioids that have not been prescribed, and prescribed opioids that are being misused.

Breastfeeding while taking prescribed pain medication (opioids) should be considered on an individual basis. Prescribed opioids during pregnancy can result in NAS, and the amount of medication required by mother and her need for the medication should be considered.

Short-term use of opioids, such as for pain control following a cesarean section, is compatible with breastfeeding. Concurrent use of other medications and medical necessity of opioids should be discussed prenatally. Transition to methadone, or decreasing the dose of prescribed medication, should also be discussed. Caution should be used for breastfeeding with codeine use since high morphine (metabolite) blood levels may occur in CYP2D6 ultra-rapid metabolizers; a death has been reported in a single case report with a mother who used codeine (11). Benefits of breastfeeding for mother and baby should be presented to the mother in an objective manner if the choice to breastfeed is ultimately her decision. Discussions should also include known information regarding breast milk for the particular medication(s); NAS symptoms which may occur after birth; and treatment for NAS with non-pharmacologic interventions, as well as the possible need for her infant to be treated with medication if her infant's symptoms cannot be controlled with non-pharmacologic methods.

Non-Opioid Drugs

There are drugs that potentiate the effects of opioids and those that can cause neurobehavioral symptoms included in the list of NAS symptoms. The following non-opioid drugs can influence NAS, and are prescribed during pregnancy or misused. In addition, polysubstance use by mother can increase the possibility and severity of NAS in the newborn (27). This list includes some commonly seen drugs with polysubstance use, and is not all-inclusive.

Alcohol

Alcohol is a nervous system depressant, and is the most common drug used and abused in the United States. Use of alcohol during pregnancy can result in fetal alcohol syndrome, partial fetal alcohol syndrome, alcohol-related neurodevelopmental disorder, and alcohol related birth defects (29). The onset of withdrawal symptoms begins at birth and may last up to 18 months or longer. Neonatal symptoms of alcohol withdrawal include hyperactive Moro reflex (startle), crying, irritability, poor suck, interrupted sleeping pattern, excessive hunger, sweating, tremors, and seizures (6).

Breastfeeding should not occur while actively drinking alcohol, and should not resume for at least several hours after drinking when the effects are no longer felt by mother. Drinking more than an occasional drink is discouraged since alcohol inhibits the release of oxytocin resulting in a decrease in letdown, decreased milk availability, and a change in the taste of breast milk causing a decrease in consumption (30). Continued moderate or excessive alcohol use can lead to a decrease in the breast milk supply and a decrease in the infant's growth. The infant may also have vomiting due the change in taste, changes in sleep, crying, and hyperactive Moro reflex.

Amphetamines

Amphetamines are synthetic psychostimulants prescribed for attention deficit hyperactivity disorder (ADHD), depression, obesity, and narcolepsy. The effects include increased heart rate, increased blood pressure, and euphoria. Amphetamines suppress appetite, reduce the sensation of fatigue, stimulate behavior, induce euphoria, and cause arousal (31). The use of amphetamines long term may cause anxiety, depression, insomnia, restlessness, paranoid psychosis, hallucinations, tremors, weight loss, and aggressive behavior.

Maternal withdrawal from amphetamines may result in hunger, mental fatigue, and mental depression, making the person become anxious, agitated, sleepy, have lucid dreams, or have suicidal ideations. Methamphetamine is far more potent than amphetamines and rarely prescribed. The byproduct of methamphetamine is amphetamines, which results in a greater amount of amphetamine crossing the blood-brain barrier, with the resultant greater effect than amphetamines.

Data available on amphetamine exposure of the infant is scarce. There are no prospective studies of withdrawal currently available. In one retrospective study done by Smith et al. (2003) using a sample of a total of 294 infants that were methamphetamine-exposed, with matching pairs which were not exposed, 49% of methamphetamine exposed infants (n=134) were reported to have symptoms of withdrawal, while four percent required pharmacologic intervention (32).

The infant's exposure to amphetamines may include drowsiness at birth, smaller head circumference, shorter length, and increased risk for ADHD in childhood (33). Using knowledge of the effects of opioid withdrawal, and effects of amphetamine exposure and withdrawal, based on timing of last maternal use, we can presume that effects of amphetamines on infants may include tremulousness and difficulty sleeping, increased muscle tone, poor feeding, and weight loss. Based on the same knowledge, withdrawal from amphetamines could result in drowsiness, poor feeding, prolonged periods of sleep, and need for feeding support, such as gavage feeding (35).

Breastfeeding is contraindicated with the illicit use of methamphetamine and amphetamines (6) and amphetamines do pass into breast milk (35). With prescribed amphetamines, there may be a decrease in serum prolactin levels, which has been reported in the few available studies (21). The breastfeeding infant should be monitored for drowsiness, weight gain, and developmental milestones after birth and during routine pediatric follow-up visits.

Barbiturates

Barbiturates are nonselective central nervous system depressants prescribed to treat anxiety, insomnia, and seizure disorders. Onset of withdrawal symptoms may begin in the newborn within the first 24 hours after birth, and can occur as late as 10 to 14 days after birth (6). If an infant is prescribed phenobarbital, duration of symptoms may be altered. Symptoms of withdrawal include irritability, disturbed sleep patterns, severe tremors, increased muscle tone, hypersensitivity to sound, excessive hunger, vomiting, loose stools, and excessive crying.

Breastfeeding while taking barbiturates may cause drowsiness, poor feeding, and sedation in the infant. The infant should be monitored for drowsiness and weight gain as well as achievement of developmental milestones after birth and during routine pediatric follow-up visits. A serum barbiturate level should be considered if the infant is very drowsy or weight gain is inadequate. With abrupt cessation of breastfeeding, startle reactions and seizures have been reported (23).

Benzodiazepines

Benzodiazepines are psychoactive drugs or tranquilizers used for treating anxiety, panic attacks, and insomnia. Benzodiazepines are also used for seizures, sedation for surgery, muscle relaxation, alcohol withdrawal, and drug-associated agitation, among others, making benzodiazepines one of the most commonly prescribed medications in the United States (36). Onset of withdrawal in the newborn occurs within hours to weeks after birth. Infants may experience hypotonia, poor suck, hypothermia, sedation, and apnea while under the influence of benzodiazepines, followed by tachypnea, tremors, hyperactive reflexes, and vomiting during withdrawal.

Breastfeeding while taking benzodiazepines may cause lethargy, drowsiness, poor feeding or laziness at the breast, and sedation in the infant (36, 37, 38). The infant should be monitored for drowsiness and weight gain, as well as achievement of developmental milestones after birth and during routine pediatric follow-up. Withdrawal symptoms, such as crying, irritability, and sleep disturbances, are possible after birth and at cessation of breastfeeding.

Caffeine

Caffeine is a central nervous system stimulant, and the most common drug ingested in the world. During pregnancy, caffeine crosses the placenta, has a prolonged half-life, and the infant has a limited ability to metabolize caffeine (39). In addition, caffeine is excreted in the urine which makes up part of the amniotic fluid. When the infant swallows the amniotic fluid, caffeine is ingested repeatedly. Under the influence of caffeine at birth, the infant may experience vomiting, bradycardia, tachypnea, fussiness, tremors, increased muscle tone, restlessness, irritability, and sleep disturbances. The long half-life and difficulty metabolizing caffeine may prolong these symptoms, which should gradually subside over the first week of life.

Breastfeeding and caffeine consumption are compatible, but generally recommended to be at a maximum of 300 mg of caffeine per day while breastfeeding a full-term healthy infant (23). Caffeine intake of more than four cups of coffee per day may cause the caffeine-sensitive infant to experience fussiness, irritability, or sleep disturbances, none of which are desired by the already sleep deprived mother.

Cocaine

Cocaine is a powerfully addictive stimulant which directly affects the brain and has been abused for over 100 years. It is an illegal substance, and also a schedule II drug that can be used as an anesthetic for some eye, ear, and throat surgeries, though not used frequently. Although an abstinence syndrome from cocaine has not been clearly identified, infants may have irritability, hyperactivity, tremors, high-pitched cry, and excessive sucking, with the onset at 48 to 72 hours after birth, and lasting up to seven days (6). Breastfeeding is not compatible with cocaine use (6, 23).

Hydroxyzine

Hydroxyzine is an antihistamine used to treat allergies, itchiness, and vomiting as well as to treat anxiety and withdrawal symptoms. Hydroxyzine can potentiate the effects of central nervous system depressants including narcotics and non-narcotic analgesics, as well as barbiturates. Under the influence of hydroxyzine, the infant may experience drowsiness or sedation. In one telephone follow-up study done by Motherisk, 10% of infants were reported by mothers to have irritability and colicky symptoms, which may also cause sleep disturbances (40). Withdrawal symptoms from the use of hydroxyzine combined with opiates may include high-pitched cry, irritability, hyperactive Moro reflex, tremors, tachypnea, tachycardia, poor feeding, and myoclonic jerks or clonic movements.

Breastfeeding while taking hydroxyzine can cause diminished milk supply in early lactation due to the antihistamine effect of decreased basal serum prolactin levels when given intravenously in high doses. However, an established breast milk supply may not be affected (23).

Nicotine

Nicotine (smoking, chewing) is a potent parasympathomimetic alkaloid, which stimulates the parasympathetic nervous system and is highly addictive. Under the influence of nicotine, the infant may experience tremors, irritability, hypertonia, and sleep disturbances (41). These symptoms have been found to be dose dependent, with an increase in symptoms following exposure to heavy smoking in the months before birth, and following maternal smoking during breastfeeding (42). These behaviors described by several authors occur immediately after birth and improve over time, suggesting the cause to be more from drug toxicity than from withdrawal, in which symptoms would increase as the remaining drug is metabolized and excreted (15).

Selective Serotonin Reuptake Inhibitors

Selective Serotonin Reuptake Inhibitors (SSRIs) are antidepressants prescribed for depression. Findings are based on small samples of infants, case reports, adverse drug reaction reports, and prospective studies linking the use of SSRIs in the third trimester of pregnancy (6). Symptoms may present within hours after birth up to several days and be the result of withdrawal or serotonin toxicity.

Following the use of SSRIs, there are individual reports of infants with one or more of the following symptoms: tremors, hyperactive Moro reflex, irritability, crying, poor suck, feeding difficulty, tachypnea, fever, sleep disturbances, myoclonic activity, and seizures (6). With a lack of randomized control studies, in addition to reports lacking evidence of infant drug levels and potential dose via breast milk, each case should be assessed individually for other potential causes of these symptoms. In the absence of opioids, most symptoms can be treated with non-pharmacological interventions. Differential diagnoses and the possibility of illness should be considered prior to assuming symptoms are the result of SSRI exposure.

Breastfeeding while taking SSRIs should be evaluated on a full individual risk:benefit evaluation, i.e., based on need, risks associated with not taking the medication, milk:plasma ratio, and potential infant dose provided through breast milk. SSRIs have been studied but lack randomized control studies (43). Multiple reviews of the literature suggest the use of SSRIs while breastfeeding is relatively safe, with paroxetine and sertraline potentially being the preferred choices with breastfeeding (44, 45). If a mother is taking a particular SSRI, and her symptoms have been in control, continuation of the same SSRI should be considered. Medication administration immediately following a breastfeeding may limit exposure for the breastfed infant. Close monitoring of maternal symptoms, as well as assessment of infant behavior and growth at routine pediatric visits is warranted. However, there is no evidence to support the routine screening of drug levels in breast milk and infant serum.

Identification of Intrauterine Drug Exposure

There is currently no standardized method to accurately identify and quantify drugs used during pregnancy. Universal drug screening is reported to be impractical, not cost effective, and biased towards women who are at an economic disadvantage, vulnerable, or of racial or ethnic minorities (5). Biological specimen testing adds to the medical costs for mother and infant and may not provide information related to the infant's medical care. Currently, the two methods used to identify drugs used during pregnancy are self-reporting and the testing of biological specimens, with the most common being urine, meconium, hair, and umbilical cord blood (31). The combined use of these two methods is likely to provide the most accurate account of drug usage during pregnancy (5).

Self-reporting provides information regarding the drug(s), amount used, and timing of usage (5). Though self-reporting is inexpensive and practical, truthfulness and memory recall can affect the accuracy of reported drug usage (46). State laws for reporting drug use during pregnancy and resultant outcomes for mother and infant impact what a woman may reveal in her self-report. The risk of charges for child abuse/neglect and potential removal of the infant from her care are two major reasons why a woman may withhold information (5).

Biological Specimens

Urine

Urine testing is the most widely used method due to the convenience of supply and time period from collection to detection. The use of urine testing is limited to the detection of recent usage, with positive results varying according to the individual drug's excretion of metabolites, type of analytical method used, and possibility of false positive or false negative results (5). Ideally, maternal urine is collected on admission and the infant's urine is collected within the first 24 hours after birth (16). Positive results are obtained when most drugs have been used within the past several days, with the exception of marijuana, which can be detected as long as 30 days after use depending on amount used (5). The turn-around time for urine toxicology results is as short as one hour making it the preferred method to screen for feasibility of breastfeeding. Urine screening tests are commonly used for the detection of alcohol, amphetamines, barbiturates, benzodiazepines, buprenorphine, cocaine, marijuana, methadone, opiates, and phencyclidine (PCP) (47).

Meconium

Meconium testing is believed to reflect the second and third trimester drug exposure during which meconium is produced within the fetus (5). Meconium is readily available in the first 24 to 48 hours after birth and is obtained through routine diaper changes. Meconium testing requires 2-3 grams of meconium and may take up to five days to obtain results if an outside lab is used (47). Due to non-uniformity of drug diffusion in meconium, it has been recommended that all meconium is collected for testing instead of a single specimen and any stool specimen that has milk stool present will most likely be rejected by the lab (16). Meconium testing should not be used to determine feasibility of breastfeeding due to the turn-around time for obtaining results. Meconium testing is limited by the availability of analytical testing in laboratories, contamination with urine, and time period of availability prior to the start of transitional stools. Meconium testing is used most commonly to detect alcohol, amphetamines, barbiturates, benzodiazepines, buprenorphine, marijuana, cocaine, nicotine, methadone, meperidine, opiates, oxycodone, phencyclidine, and tramadol (47).

Hair

Hair testing reflects drug use over a longer period of time, but may be limited by the availability of analytical testing in laboratories, the amount of hair needed, concern for cosmetic appearance, chemicals used on the hair, and beliefs about hair cutting for infants (5). Turn-around time for hair testing can be done in as little as 24 hours for a negative result and requires an additional three to five days to confirm drug identification for a positive test (47). Initiation of breastfeeding within the first hours after birth is impossible if hair testing is used to determine feasibility of breastfeeding. Use of hair for drug testing is not commonly used in the clinical setting for newborns. Hair testing is used most commonly to detect amphetamines, barbiturates, benzodiazepines, buprenorphine, cocaine, marijuana, methadone, nicotine, opiates, and phencyclidine (47).

Umbilical Cord

The umbilical cord can also be used to detect drugs used during pregnancy and is available at delivery (5). Toxicology testing of the umbilical cord is limited by the availability of analytical testing in laboratories, availability of the specimen only after birth, and turn-around time for results. With overnight shipping, turn-around time for negative test results is generally the

102

same day the specimen is received, with an additional 24 to 48 hours required for presumed positive results in order to complete the identification of drugs (47). Initiation of breastfeeding within the first hours after birth is impossible if umbilical cord testing is used to determine feasibility of breastfeeding. The umbilical cord can be used to detect alcohol, amphetamines, barbiturates, benzodiazepines, buprenorphine, cannabinoids, cocaine, methadone, meperidine, opiates, oxycodone, phencyclidine, and tramadol (47).

Breast Milk

Breast milk availability in the first couple days after childbirth may limit breast milk testing since the test requires about 10 mL of breast milk and the priority of the use of breast milk is to provide it to the infant (47). Results are obtained in 24 hours for negative specimens, with an additional two to three days for positive specimens. Toxicology testing of breast milk is limited by the availability of analytical testing in laboratories, specimen availability in the first days after birth, skill needed to obtain the specimen, and turn-around time for results. Breast milk testing should not be used to determine feasibility of breastfeeding initiation due to the 24-hour delay in turn-around time. Breast milk testing is most commonly used to detect alcohol, amphetamines, barbiturates, benzodiazepines, buprenorphine, cocaine, marijuana, methadone, meperidine, nicotine, opiates, oxycodone, phencyclidine, and tramadol (47).

Presentation of NAS

The onset of NAS can begin as early as right after birth and progress as the infant is able to metabolize and eliminate the prescribed medication or illicit drug, with some symptoms occasionally lasting through most of the first year after birth. The onset of withdrawal symptoms varies for different drugs and is affected by factors including the drug type, dose, half-life, route of administration, last maternal dose, frequency of use, length of exposure, infant metabolism, and gestational age. Prior to assuming NAS symptoms are related to opioid withdrawal, other more serious diagnoses should be ruled out. Examples of diagnoses that should be investigated include hypoglycemia (tremors, poor feeding, seizures), hypocalcemia (tachypnea, poor feeding, tremors, seizures), infection (crying, irritability, poor feeding, vomiting, diarrhea), hyperthyroidism (irritability, difficulty sleeping, vomiting, diarrhea), and hypoxic-ischemic encephalopathy (increased muscle tone, poor feeding, irritability, crying, seizures).

Symptoms present as disturbances in the central nervous system (tremors, increased muscle tone, high-pitched crying), gastrointestinal system (poor feeding, vomiting, loose stools), and vasomotor/respiratory system (tachypnea, fever, sneezing). The number and severity of symptoms represent the lack of self-regulation in the infant resulting from the effects of disturbances between the parasympathetic and sympathetic nervous systems. The display of symptoms is unique to each newborn infant.

Mother and Infant

Education should begin prenatally and continue throughout the pregnancy, post-partum period, and beyond. Prenatal care should include education on breastfeeding, skin-to-skin care, and parenting. Discussion and evaluation for feasibility of breastfeeding should begin prenatally with reassessment at delivery. Early initiation of breastfeeding right after delivery is facilitated using skin-to-skin care. Development of parenting skills, and access to available community resources, empowers the new mother to 1) care for herself and her baby, and 2) develop mutual regulation for herself and her infant by reading her infant's cue and responding appropriately.

Mother's presence and involvement in the care of her infant with NAS has been shown to decrease the severity of symptoms, need for pharmacological treatment, length of treatment, and amount of medication administered (48). Mother-infant attachment, or bonding, results from close proximity enabling mother to respond to her infant's cues by touching, holding, feeding, looking at, and talking to her baby. Ideally, mother and infant rooming together provides the maximum opportunity to develop the mother-infant attachment through interactions with each other. If mother is unable to care for her baby due to difficult birth, C-section, or illness, then her partner, a family member, or friend should be present to assist her. If no one is able to stay with mother, nursery care can be provided until mother is able to care for her own baby.

External regulation may be needed when NAS symptoms are present. The mother is the optimal person to respond to her infant's cues and provide this regulation. Responses to her infant can assist the infant to tolerate symptoms and decrease the severity of NAS. Keeping the mother and infant together allows the mother to learn her baby's cues and respond immediately. Health care providers can provide education regarding methods to assist the mother and infant through the withdrawal period including environmental controls and non-pharmacologic interventions.

Breastfeeding, when determined to be feasible, can also assist the infant through the withdrawal period. The act of breastfeeding allows for close interactions between the mother and her infant, and this closeness may provide added comfort for the infant. Studies on methadone or buprenorphine amounts found in breast milk confirm that the amounts in breast milk are not high enough to provide treatment for NAS (27, 49, 50).

Care of the Infant with NAS Symptoms

Observation for symptoms of NAS begins right after birth, with the first assessment done by two hours of age. Non-pharmacological interventions should begin immediately after birth to reduce the number and severity of symptoms. Between 55 to 94% of opioid-exposed infants require pharmacological treatment, in addition to the continued use of non-pharmacological interventions (6). Assessment of symptoms is done by nursing staff every three to four hours during the hospital stay. Length of hospital stay is related to the type of substance exposure, display of NAS symptoms, and requirements for pharmacological treatment.

Assessment of NAS

Multiple tools exist for the assessment of NAS, including the modified Finnegan scoring tool, Lipsitz Neonatal Drug Withdrawal Scoring System, Neonatal Narcotic Withdrawal Index, Neonatal Withdrawal Inventory, and the Ostrea tool. The most commonly used tool is the modified Finnegan tool derived from the original Finnegan Neonatal Abstinence Score developed in 1975 (51, 52). Many versions of the modified Finnegan tool are in use today since various healthcare providers have adjusted the definitions of the symptoms and the related numeric scores. These tools were originally developed to assess for symptoms of opiate withdrawal but are currently being used for polysubstance withdrawal. Though symptoms may have seemingly objective definitions, the introduction of subjective information can alter scores. Regardless of the tool chosen, the accuracy of the tool is improved by all persons using the tool in the same manner. Inter-rater reliability testing improves the accuracy of the tool's use, and allows providers to base pharmacological treatment on the NAS scores.

Treatment of NAS

Environmental and non-pharmacological interventions should begin immediately following birth by placing the infant skin-to-skin with mother. The environment should be assessed for stimuli that can disturb the infant, and efforts should be made to remove the stimuli (52). Environmental stimuli can be a variety of things that stimulate the infant's senses. Sight is stimulated by bright lights and visual sights in the immediate environment, including the human face. Dimming the lights and limiting visual stimuli to just the faces of parents may help to decrease the infant's irritability. Eliminate strong smells, such as tobacco smoke and perfumes, and replace with the mother's scent and the smell of her breasts. Audio stimuli, such as phone tones, door bells, and TV volume, should be minimized, and speaking should be in a quiet voice. The infant that is sensitive to touch can be held skin-to-skin or swaddled with a blanket. If tolerated, the infant may relax with massage or cuddling. Eliminate disturbing movements, such as bouncing or abrupt movements. Continuous evaluation of how external stimuli affect the infant is needed as the infant excretes the remaining drug(s) and metabolite(s) and the symptoms of NAS increase. Provide support for the parents, and encourage rooming-in for support of breastfeeding and mother-infant attachment. Clustering cares together around feeding times will help to avoid disrupting the sleeping infant.

In general, neonatal withdrawal from a drug should be treated with the same drug, or one in the same classification, e.g., opiate withdrawal treated with morphine. Pharmacological treatment is initiated when NAS scores rise to a predetermined number or the infant's symptoms result in the inability to eat, sleep, and grow. Multiple medications have been used for treatment of NAS including, but not limited to, morphine, methadone, phenobarbital, and benzodiazepines. Non-pharmacological interventions should be continued to aid in decreasing the infant's symptoms and severity, while decreasing the need for medication, the total amount of medication required, and hospital length of stay.

The substance-exposed infant without medical complications is ideally cared for in an environment that allows mother to stay with her baby whenever possible (53). Separation of mother from her infant increases the stress on the family, which may already be stressed. Mothers may experience feelings of guilt when their infant shows symptoms of NAS, and separation from their infant may leave them feeling inadequate and helpless to care for her own child. Keeping mothers and infants together allows the mother to learn her own infant's cues and how to best care for her infant. Keeping them together empowers mothers to care for their own infants in the hospital and at home, which has been shown to improve outcomes such as decreased length of stay and decreased need for medication (54).

Long-Term Infant Outcomes of Intrauterine Drug Exposure

Long-term outcomes of intrauterine drug exposure have been reviewed for some drugs and illicit substances, many of which have no clear-cut answer. Outcomes that have been reviewed or studied include growth, behavior, development, and language (5). These outcomes are in need of further research with controls for health and environment. When considering the effects of individual substances, it is difficult to attribute a specific symptom to a specific substance due to non-specificity and overlapping of symptoms. The effects of individual substances must be considered to appreciate the

106

complexities and clinical status of the drug-exposed infant (17) (see Table 8-3 Observed Effects of Substance Abuse in the Newborn). The systematic review of literature and meta-analysis by Baldacchino, Arbuckle, Petrie, and McCowan in 2104, found "no significant impairments in cognitive, psychomotor or observed behavioral outcomes for chronic intrauterine exposed infant and pre-school children, although in all domains there is a trend toward poor outcomes in infants/children of opioid using mothers" (p. 8) (55) . Their study excluded polysubstance use (55) and plausible confusion of NAS neurobehavior outcomes and other neonatal presentations of opioid withdrawal (12) due to the stringent inclusion criteria which limited the number of studies analyzed to four (55).

Breastfeeding

There are well-known benefits from breastfeeding for both mother and infant. Examples of maternal benefits include the reduced risk of breast, uterine and ovarian cancers and osteoporosis, delayed ovulation from frequent breastfeeding resulting in natural child-spacing, less postpartum anxiety and depression, earlier return to pre-pregnant weight, and improved health related to self-care. Examples of benefits for the infant include the unique food source for each individual infant with essential nutrients, increased resistance to infection (e.g. respiratory infection, vomiting, diarrhea) in the early months from maternal antibodies in breast milk, improved cognitive ability, decreased risk of developing allergies, protection from obesity, and decreased risk of sudden infant death syndrome. There are additional benefits for the drug-dependent woman and her infant from breastfeeding and mother's milk, especially for those at risk for health and developmental issues, e.g., promotion of bonding; decreased symptoms of NAS from the act of breastfeeding; decreased need for medication; and decreased length of hospital stay (48). The inclusion of prenatal planning in preparation for breastfeeding and parenting, as well as planned postpartum and pediatric follow-up after discharge from the hospital is strongly recommended.

Education to Promote Breastfeeding

Breastfeeding education should begin during prenatal care and continue during hospitalization for delivery. After discharge, breastfeeding education should continue during the infant's primary care provider visits until the infant weans from the breast. Prenatal and postpartum education should include abstaining from the use of illicit substances, use of prescription medication as prescribed, and instructions for what to do in the event of relapse to drug or alcohol use when breastfeeding. Include in mother's education when to provide previously stored breast milk or formula to her infant and in what situations breastfeeding is contraindicated. Education on formula use and preparation, as well as bottle use, should be provided for times when stored breast milk is not available. It is important for the mother to contact her health care provider to be evaluated for resumption of breastfeeding. Before resumption of breastfeeding, each situation should be evaluated to determine if risks to the infant outweigh the benefits of breastfeeding.

The Decision to Breastfeed

Pregnant women choose to breastfeed because they want to provide the ideal nutrition for their infants. Women who use or misuse drugs choose to breastfeed for the same reason, but due to their substance use or misuse, they have other obstacles to consider, such as additional hospital policies applied to any women with a history of substance use or misuse, with or without a prescription (48). The woman with substance use/misuse may be required to have a negative toxicology screen, a negative toxicology screen on her infant after birth, be actively involved in a drug treatment program or followed by a community physician in the case of buprenorphine, and have planned follow-up care for herself and her infant prior to discharge (48). In addition, breastfeeding the infant with symptoms of NAS can be difficult; however, all the effort put into breastfeeding result in the known benefits for mother and infant as well as comfort for the infant from the act of breastfeeding.

An International Board Certified Lactation Consultant (IBCLC) is in the ideal position to assist the new mother to be successful at breastfeeding using the knowledge of helping a woman to be successful at breastfeeding and the knowledge of NAS. The IBCLC can participate in a multidisciplinary health care team to determine the safety, benefits, and contraindications in the setting of substance use during pregnancy. The IBCLC may be involved in determining if breastfeeding is feasible but the IBCLC is not responsible for making medical decisions unless he / she is also a licensed healthcare provider (physician, nurse practitioner, physician assistant).

Before the initiation of breastfeeding, all mother-infant dyads should be evaluated to determine their individual situation and compatibility with breastfeeding. All factors should be considered when evaluating for compatibility (see Table 8.4 Factors to Consider in Evaluating Breastfeeding Compatibility), especially prenatal information related to substance use, involvement in treatment, and relapses, which should all be communicated to the healthcare team. Ideally, written maternal consent should be obtained to enable communication between all of mother's and infant's care providers, thereby creating a team approach to prenatal and postnatal healthcare management.

Assessing for Readiness to Breastfeed

There are six behavioral states for infants: quiet sleep, active sleep, drowsy, quiet alert, active alert, and crying (56). Each state has behavioral characteristics specific to that state, including body activity, eye movements, facial movements, breathing pattern, and level of response to external and internal stimuli. Change from one behavioral state to another is generally a gradual process which is affected by the infant's wellbeing, the environment, and the infant's caregiver. Infants with poor state control may go from quiet sleep to crying when disturbed by symptoms of NAS, the environment, or the caregiver (20).

The quiet alert state is the ideal behavioral state for breastfeeding and may be difficult to maintain in the infant experiencing symptoms of NAS. Non-pharmacological interventions are the first-line treatment to attain, maintain, and sustain the quiet alert state. Prepare for breastfeeding by decreasing external stimuli in the environment. Dimming lighting, reducing audio volumes including voice, and minimizing movement such as rocking and bouncing, all result in less stimulation for the infant. Breastfeeding should begin with skin-to-skin by holding the sleeping infant near the breast with the infant's hands placed on each side of the breast and providing open access for latching. Provide minimal stimuli and allow the infant to awaken at the breast.

Positioning the infant at the breast may become more difficult with increased muscle tone and rapid rooting. Infants use their hands to locate the nipple and these hands may get in the way as they attempt to get the nipple into their mouth. Swaddling the infant with the hands and arms down may seem like it would remove the hands and facilitate latching, however, this may confuse the infant. Colson (2012) described the use of biological nursing to promote successful breastfeeding and the principles of skin-to-skin, infant lying prone on mother, and mother lying back at rest can be used to promote mother-centered breastfeeding (57). As symptoms of NAS increase, it may be necessary to lead the infant to the breast face-first and wrap the arms and hands around the breast to assist the infant in latching on to the breast. Genna and Barak (2010) described how an infant uses the hands to locate, move, and shape the nipple in the process of latching on to the breast (58). A hands-off approach by healthcare providers can be used with reassurance to mother and education on how her infant uses primitive neonatal reflexes to reach the breast and complete a successful breastfeeding. The infant with uncoordinated suck and swallow may have difficulty latching on and maintaining the latch. Early breastfeeding initiation and frequent feedings in the first few days improve the infant's breastfeeding ability when increasing symptoms develop.

Mother and infant rooming together provides for more opportunities for the mother to learn her infant's cues. For example, the infant that is irritable and crying may be interpreted as being hungry, and the mother may make frequent attempts to breastfeed with repeated failures, resulting in a decrease in the mother's confidence to breastfeed or mother her own infant. If irritability and crying is interpreted as pain, the mother may attribute the cause to gas or stomach cramping, resulting in her request for medication for gas to minimize her infant's discomfort. When the infant escalates to the crying state, the infant's ability to breastfeed is reduced unless mother is taught how to calm her baby. Removal of the infant from mother may undermine her confidence in her own ability to breastfeed her infant. When the infant is crying or rooting with the head shaking left to right, gravity from the laid-back position can help keep the infant's face toward the breast. Ultimately, the number-one priority is getting the breast milk to the infant; therefore, breast pumping and bottle feeding mother's milk may be necessary until symptoms of NAS are in better control. This should be a temporary fix, and attempts at breastfeeding should continue with the goal of feeding at the breast for all feedings.

Successful Breastfeeding

Early confirmation of the compatibility of breastfeeding with the individual woman's situation allows for early initiation of breastfeeding. Ideally, the healthy full-term or preterm infant is placed on mother's chest / abdomen skin-to-skin immediately after birth. Achieving the best behavioral state for successful breastfeeding, quiet alert, is ideal for the infant to latch to the breast and transfer milk. Early and frequent breastfeedings assist in establishing breast milk supply, improves the infant's ability to breastfeed before NAS symptoms interfere, and allows the mother to develop some confidence in her infant's ability to latch and suckle, as well as her own ability to read her infant's cues and provide an adequate supply of breast milk.

Breastfeeding During Symptom Escalation

Breastfeeding the infant with NAS becomes a challenge when the symptoms increase in number and severity. Providing anticipatory education for mother may assist her through the symptom escalation. Earlier successes with breastfeeding provide an advantage for continued breastfeeding during escalation if the infant is able to continue to latch and suckle. Interpretation of the infant's behavioral state and interventions to achieve the quiet-alert state, known to be most successful for breastfeeding, also improve breastfeeding outcomes.

Weaning

Gradual weaning from the breast occurs naturally in the older infant. Initially, breast milk is the infant's complete diet, and as the infant grows, solids are added to the diet. Currently, there is a lack of research on breast milk levels of methadone and buprenorphine and related effects in the older infant. Single reports found in the literature have reported withdrawal symptoms with a rapid or abrupt weaning from breast milk; however, adequate detail is lacking to determine the frequency of withdrawal. The recommendation is for gradual weaning from breast milk until further research is available.

Table 8.1 Symptoms of Neonatal Opioid Withdrawal

High-pitched cry	Poor feeding
Excessive irritability	Vomiting
Hyperactive Moro reflex	Loose stools
Increased muscle tone	Failure to thrive
Excoriation	Sweating
Interrupted sleep-wake cycles	Sneezing
Tremors disturbed/undisturbed	Nasal stuffiness
Seizures	Yawning
Elevated temperature	Tachypnea

Table 8.2 Opiate Duration of Action and Half-Life

Drug	Duration of Action	Average Half-Life of Elimination
Codeine	4 to 6 hours	3 to 4 hours
Heroin	3 to 4 hours	2 to 6 minutes; metabolite 6 hours
Hydrocodone	4 to 8 hours	3.8 hours
Hydromorphone	3 to 4 hours	2.4 hours
Meperidine	2 to 4 hours	2 to 5 hours; metabolite 15 to 30 hours
Morphine	4 hours	1.5 to 3 hours
Oxycodone	3 to 5 hours	3 to 4 hours (immediate release) 4 to 6 hours (controlled release)

Table 8.3 Observed Effects of Substance Abuse in the Newborn

Reprinted with revisions with permission. Jansson, L.M. & Velez, M. (2011). Infants of drug-dependent mothers. Pediatrics in Review, 32(1), 5-13.

	Nicotine	Alcohol	Marijuana	Cocaine	PCP	Opioids	Meth-amphetamine	Benzo-diazepines
Prematurity	Yes	Yes	No	Yes	No	Yes/No	Yes/No	Yes
Low Birth Weight	Yes	Yes	Yes/No	Yes	No	Yes/No	Yes	Yes
Neuro-behavioral Symptoms	Yes	Yes	Yes	Yes	Yes	Yes	Yes	Yes
NAS	Yes	Yes	No	No?	Yes	Yes/No	Yes?	Yes
Congenital Mal-formations	Yes/No	Yes	No?	Yes/No	No	Yes/No	Yes?	Yes/No

Yes/No=both have been reported, ?=controversial, NAS=neonatal abstinence syndrome,

PCP=phencyclidine

Table 8.4 Factors to Consider in Evaluating Breastfeeding Compatibility

Current substance use or misuse
History of substance use or misuse
Treatment with methadone or buprenorphine
Medical status
Psychiatric status
Maternal need for other medications
Infant's current health status
Evaluation of NAS and impact on infant's ability to breastfeed
Maternal family support –presence, absence, adequacy
Community support system – presence, absence, adequacy
Plans for postpartum follow-up care
Maintenance treatment for substance use
Psychiatric care if warranted
Pediatric follow-up care

Chapter 9: Treatment Drugs

Amy C. Luo

I was the senior resident in peds on call at the peds ER in Chicago's Cook County. At about 3 AM, the triage nurse, rather a slow creature, walked patiently to my exam room and said quietly: "Dr. R., there is a patient who is hardly breathing." Startled, I jumped and ran out to see the kid, about one week of age, indeed was hardly breathing—cold, and very bradycardic. We rushed the kid to the peds ward and did CPR. As I stabilized the baby on a vent, I began a detailed exam, and noted the pin-point-pupil. Morphine effect? Something hit me. I asked the mom about what happened—she did not say much. I then said that if she did not tell me the truth, her baby would probably die soon. Then I learned that the mom had gone home earlier that week from the County OB ward. Her prenatal and natal histories were "nothing remarkable." But after I said again that she was not telling me more details, she said that she added a spoon full of heroin into the baby formula and fed the baby, because the baby was showing signs of withdrawal (which she recognized based on her experience) and decided to treat the condition herself. When the baby gradually stopped breathing, she brought the baby to the hospital.

We reversed the heroin effect with naltrexone, the kid was extubated the same day, and went home after the social service department registered her for follow-up.

(Name withheld by request; used with permission)

What are some options for managing dependence in pregnant and breastfeeding women? Will these medications affect the fetus or the breastfeeding infant? This chapter lists treatment options to aid healthcare providers to select compatible and effective strategies.

Definitions of Pregnancy and Breastfeeding Recommendations (1, 2)

Pregnancy

- **Compatible** - The human pregnancy experience is adequate to demonstrate that the embryo-fetal risk is very low or nonexistent.

- **No (Limited) Human Data - Animal Data Suggests Low Risk** - Either there is no human pregnancy experience or the few pregnancy exposures have not been associated with developmental toxicity. The drug <u>does not</u> cause developmental toxicity in all animal species studied at doses ≤ 10 times the human dose based on body surface area or area under the plasma concentration vs. time curve.

- **Limited Human Data - Animal Data Suggest Moderate Risk** - Either there is no human pregnancy experience or the few pregnancy exposures have not been associated with developmental toxicity. The drug <u>causes</u> developmental toxicity in one animal species at doses ≤ 10 times the human dose based on body surface area or area under the plasma concentration vs. time curve.

- **No (Limited) Human Data - No Relevant Animal Data** - There is no human or animal pregnancy data, or the human pregnancy experience, that may or may not include the First Trimester, is limited. The risk in pregnancy cannot be assessed.

Breastfeeding

- **No (Limited) Human Data - Probably Compatible** - Either there is no human data or the human data are limited. The available data suggest that the drug does not represent a significant risk to a nursing infant.

- **No (Limited) Human Data - Potential Toxicity** - Either there is no human data or the human data are limited. The characteristics of the drug suggest that it could represent a clinically significant risk to a nursing infant. Breastfeeding is not recommended.

Treatment Drugs

Disulfiram (3)

Pregnancy: Limited Human Data - No Relevant Animal Data
Congenital defects have been reported.
Consider this: These defects may be related to alcohol exposure.

Breastfeeding: No Human Data - Potential Toxicity
Excretion into breastmilk is expected. However, effects of exposure to nursing infants are unknown.

Although the long-term effectiveness of disulfiram has not been established in the prevention of alcoholism, it is a useful adjunct to psychotherapy. Disulfiram is the most widely used agent for conditioned aversion in alcoholics.

Methadone (4, 5)

Pregnancy: Human Data Suggest Risk
No congenital defects observed.
Consider this: Patients may consume a wide variety of drugs, not possible to distinguish effects of methadone from effects of other agents. Withdrawal symptoms and low birth weight are the main concerns.

Breastfeeding: Limited Human Data - Probably Compatible
Excretion into breastmilk is negligible. No adverse effects of the exposure were observed during breastfeeding or during weaning.

Methadone is indicated for the management of moderate to severe pain when a continuous, around-the-clock opioid analgesic is needed for an extended period of time. It should not be used as an as-needed analgesic, for pain that is mild or not expected to persist, for acute pain, and / or for postoperative pain. The pharmacokinetic properties of methadone and the high inter-patient variability in absorption, metabolism, and relative analgesic potency of methadone necessitate a cautious and individualized approach to prescribing. Special attention is required during treatment initiation, during conversion from one opioid to another, and during dose titration. When determining the initial methadone dose for chronic pain management, the following factors should be considered: total daily dose, potency, and prior opioid the patient has been taking previously; degree of opioid experience and opioid tolerance; general medical condition; concurrent medication; and type and severity of pain.

Methadone is also indicated for detoxification treatment of opioid addiction (heroin or other morphine-like drugs) and for maintenance treatment of opioid addiction in conjunction with appropriate social and medical services. In either case, methadone shall be dispensed only by certified opioid treatment programs as stipulated in 42 Code of Federal Regulations (CFR) Section 8.12.

Injectable methadone is only approved for use in the temporary treatment of opioid dependence in hospitalized patients unable to take oral medication; it is not approved for outpatient use.

Buprenorphine / Naloxone (6)

Pregnancy: Limited Human Data - Animal Data Suggest Low Risk
No congenital defects in one pregnancy case. Weak neonatal withdrawal symptoms were observed.
Consider this: There are more published human pregnancy experiences for

other narcotic analgesics, so buprenorphine is not the preferred narcotic analgesic during pregnancy.

Breastfeeding: Limited Human Data - Potential Toxicity
Excreted into human milk. No withdrawal symptoms in the infant were observed.
Consider this: Decreased nursing and milk ingestion will result in lower weight gain.

Buprenorphine and naloxone sublingual (SL) film and buprenorphine and naloxone SL tablets are indicated for induction therapy for patients dependent on heroin or other short-acting opioids. Induction should be started only after objective signs of moderate withdrawal appear and at least six hours following the last opioid dose. For patients dependent on methadone or long-acting opioids, buprenorphine monotherapy is recommended for induction.

Buprenorphine and naloxone SL film, SL tablets, and buccal film are indicated for the maintenance treatment of opioid dependence as part of a complete treatment plan to include counseling and psychosocial support. Prescription use of the product is limited to prescribers who meet certain qualifying requirements and have notified the Secretary of Health and Human Services (HHS) of their intent to prescribe the product. Buprenorphine and naloxone SL tablets are effective in reducing craving and increasing the incidence of negative opioid urine samples and subject retention.

Sublingual buprenorphine and naloxone should be considered a regimen of choice for the treatment of opioid maintenance therapy and is particularly useful in the primary care office-based setting. Naloxone has no effect on buprenorphine efficacy, and withdrawal symptoms do not occur when tablets are used properly; however, full naloxone-antagonist effects occur if SL tablets are dissolved in water and injected, thus minimizing abuse and misuse. The ceiling effect of buprenorphine reduces the severity of overdose and limits abuse liability. Studies have demonstrated a significant reduction in opioid craving and high retention of opioid-dependent subjects during therapy.

Naloxone (7)

Pregnancy: Compatible
Naloxone does not have respiratory depressive actions or other narcotic properties. Naloxone crosses the placenta. Naloxone can safely be given to newborns within a few minutes of delivery. Naloxone may enhance fetal asphyxia, leading to fatal respiratory failure. Thus, naloxone should not be

given to the mother just before delivery or to newborns, unless narcotic toxicity is evident.

Breastfeeding: No Human Data - Probably Compatible
No data are available.

Naloxone is indicated for partial or complete reversal of opioid depression induced by natural or synthetic opioids, such as methadone, and certain mixed agonist-antagonist analgesics, including nalbuphine, pentazocine, butorphanol, and cyclazocine. The clinical response to naloxone may be incomplete or higher doses may be required for respiratory depression caused by partial agonists or mixed agonist/antagonists, such as buprenorphine or pentazocine.

Naloxone injection is also indicated for the diagnosis of known or suspected acute opioid overdose.

Naloxone may be useful as adjunctive therapy for the management of septic shock; however, the optimal dose and treatment regimen have not been established. In some cases of septic shock, naloxone use has been associated with a rise in blood pressure lasting for several hours, but this pressor response has not been shown to improve patient survival. Caution is advised when using naloxone for septic shock, particularly among patients with underlying pain or previously treated with opioid therapy, as opioid tolerance may have developed.

Naloxone Hydrochloride Injection (TM) is a hand-held auto-injector product intended for the emergency treatment of known or suspected opioid overdose. The auto-injector is equipped with an electronic voice instruction system to assist caregivers with administration.

Naltrexone (8)

Pregnancy: Limited Human Data - Animal Data Suggest Moderate Risk
No congenital defects noted in animal studies.
Consider this: Naltrexone is likely to cross the placenta and alter some opioid receptors in the brain. Long lasting effects include decreased effectiveness of morphine analgesia in those exposed.

Breastfeeding: Limited Human Data - Probably Compatible
Excreted into breastmilk. No adverse effects were observed in one case report.

The extended-release injectable formulation of naltrexone is indicated for the treatment of alcohol dependence in patients who are able to abstain from alcohol in an outpatient setting before initiation of naltrexone treatment. It is also indicated for the prevention of relapse to opioid dependence following opioid detoxification.

While pretreatment with oral naltrexone is not required, patients must be opioid-free and should not be actively drinking alcohol at the time of initial administration. While oral naltrexone hydrochloride is dosed once daily, the extended-release naltrexone injection is administered intramuscularly once a month. Naltrexone therapy should include psychosocial support as part of a comprehensive management program for both indications.

Naltrexone is an effective adjunctive treatment in individuals with alcohol dependence. Combined with supportive therapy, it is useful in decreasing the craving for alcohol and particularly useful in preventing alcohol relapse once intake of alcohol occurs.

Naltrexone is an effective narcotic antagonist in the management of opiate addiction. The drug is not a treatment for addiction, but rather an adjunct to social and psychological assistance in rehabilitation. Three types of patients seem well suited for naltrexone therapy: adolescent (short-term) heroin users, abstinent addicts at risk (e.g., released prisoners), and recently detoxified methadone patients. Freshly detoxified, heroin-dependent individuals have not been demonstrated to be good choices for naltrexone therapy due to poor motivation and non-compliance.

Chapter 10: Counseling

Amy C. Luo; Frank J. Nice

I got a call from a court representative stating that a judge had ordered that a mother whose xxxth baby was also removed from her and placed in foster care wanted to pump and provide her breast milk for her baby. She had a WIC pump and they wanted assessment and education to be provided. I was fearful, as I did not want to "assure" anyone that this mom would stay clean and provide safe milk. At the same time, I did want to inform her of the dangers her baby might face if she did provide drug-laced milk. I had been trained using the interventions of the "4P's Plus© Screen for Substance Use in Pregnancy," and decided to use a similar format.

I met her at the location arranged for her to visit her baby (a 3rd party location, so she would not be able to identify the foster mom). After her visit with her baby, we sat and talked, she assured me she was not using any drugs. I explained to her it was "court ordered" that I must discuss what MIGHT happen if she did provide her baby her milk after using drugs. I then proceeded to review each drug that she had a history of using (repeatedly saying I believed her that she was not using, but that she needed to know what might happen to her baby is she did and provided her milk to be given to her baby). I had the book *Medications and Mothers' Milk*, with sticky notes on each drug. I reviewed the L1-L5 risk description and then went to each drug and read the risks to her baby. I then reviewed the way to pump and store her milk. We parted with her still saying she did not use drugs. However, I learned later that she never took her milk for her baby during visits, and she had returned the breast pump to WIC many months later (she never regained custody if her baby).

Later on, I learned from WIC that she had ANOTHER baby—and this time was "clean and sober" and breastfed! This was not the result of my intervention alone, I am sure. We had a team of people interacting with this mom with consistent messaging prenatally with the Comprehensive Perinatal Services Program of California and WIC, in the hospital, and postpartum with a Public Health Nurse and WIC. I was relieved her previous baby was not additionally exposed after birth…and that the next one had a better start in life!

Counseling Addendum: The above case is not about Brianna, but in her interview, Brianna mentioned that she had been seeing an out-of-pocket counselor, but could not afford to keep doing so. *"I had been going on my own*

120

[to see an addiction counselor]… and I stopped doing that, right around the time that I got pregnant, because of the money….the drive, the gas, the time…

(Continued in Chapter 11)

All healthcare professionals should never give up or allow our patients to ever give up.

Figure 10.1 Never Give Up!

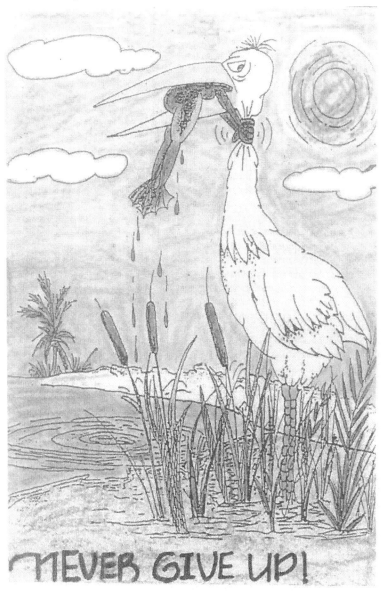

Introduction

The Academy of Managed Care Pharmacy (AMCP) described the Indian Health Service (IHS) as an influencer, whose innovative practice changed the delivery of pharmaceutical care around the world. The IHS method of prescription counseling utilizes open-ended questions to direct a dialogue that covers three major areas of understanding: (1, 2)

1. Why do you take this medication?

2. How did the doctor tell you to take the medication? (How do you take it?)

    a. Use other open-ended questions to break up the "How" discussion?
    e.g., "What does three times a day mean to you?"

3. What did the doctor tell you to expect? (What kind of problems are you having?)

Obviously, medical providers do not provide directions for patients to use substances recreationally under normal circumstances. Therefore, it is necessary to modify the counseling questions listed above. The questions in parenthesis may be a good place to start.

Talking With Patients

Keep in mind that our patients may be anxious, worried, distressed, and / or confused. These emotions can be extreme when the substances in question are for recreational use. Some tips to remember include:

- **Technical words or jargon** (3)
  It may be natural to use "physician-speak," but going beyond necessary technical terms to write in jargon can cause misunderstanding or alienation. To our patients, special terms can be difficult or meaningless. If a technical word must be used, define it for the patient.

- **Unnecessary details**
  Reduce confusion or information overload by reducing information covered. Use simple vocabulary and short sentences. Make no more than two or three key points for each topic.

- **Acronyms**
  If an acronym must be used, explain the meaning the first time you use it.

- **"Teach-Back" method**
  Avoid asking patients, "Do you understand?" Most will say they do even when they are confused. Instead say "I want to make sure I did a good job teaching you. Tell me how you are going to do this when you get home." The "Teach-Back" method has been validated to improve recall and participation in the treatment plan.

- **Pictures** (4)
  Consider "The Falling Man," by photographer Richard Drew: A man falling from the North Tower of the World Trade Center during the September 11 attacks in New York City. This image appeared as a full spread on The New York Times on September 12th, 2001. Beyond the graphic composition, the Falling Man looks composed. It is a horrific moment, but there is calmness to the image. Readers across the country cried that this image was offensive, that it should have never been published. As a result, it disappeared from sight very quickly. However, a film was later made about this photograph. "What was it about this image that Americans found so distasteful?" asked the film director, Henry Singer. "The only way we can understand the world — and part of the world is the horror of the world—is to be a witness to these images." A picture is worth a thousand words. Illustrations convey instructions better than words.

- **Talk with family members** (5)
  Enlist the aid of a family member or a friend if you think your patient may have low health literacy. In a situation where patients are using recreational substances, patients may have closed communication with family members and friends, or do not have support at all. Consider reaching out to a counseling service or home health service, and help patients enroll in a support group.

Helping Patients Set Goals

Goal setting should be patient-directed, specific, and set around a specific measurable timeframe. Healthcare providers can utilize these two tools to achieve patient-centered goal setting.

- **Ultra-Brief Personal Action Plan** (UB-PAP) (6)
  Allows clinicians to support patient self-management.
  Encourages the patient to develop his or her behavior specific action plan.

- **Motivational Interviewing** (MI) (7, 8)
  Originally developed for addiction counseling.
  Guided approach that creates a safe environment by avoiding

shaming and blaming the patient.
Follows the "READS" principles:

- **R**oll with resistance

  - [Patient] I do not want to stop drinking. As I said, I do not have a drinking problem. I want to drink when I feel like it.
    [Healthcare Provider (HCP)] Others may think you have a problem, but you don't.
    [Patient] That's right, my mother thinks that I have a problem, but she's wrong.

- **E**xpress empathy

  - [Patient] I am so tired, but I cannot even sleep, so I drink some wine.
    [HCP] You drink wine to help you sleep.
    [Patient] When I wake up, it is too late already. Yesterday my boss fired me.
    [HCP] So you're concerned about not having a job.
    [Patient] …but I do not have a drinking problem.

- **A**void argumentation

  - [Patient] I do not want to stop drinking. As I said, I do not have a drinking problem. I want to drink when I feel like it.
    [HCP] **But, I think it is clear that drinking has caused your problems.**
    [Patient] You do not have the right to judge me. You don't understand me.

- **D**evelop discrepancy

  - [Patient] I enjoy having some drinks with my friends, that's all. Drinking helps me relax and have fun. I think that I deserve that for a change.
    [HCP] So drinking has some good things for you, now tell me about the not-so-good things you have experienced because of drinking.
    [Patient] Well, as I said, I lost my job because of my drinking problem, and I often feel sick.

- Support self-efficacy
  - [Patient] I am wondering if you can help me. I have failed many times.
    [HCP] I don't think you have failed because you are still here, hoping things can be better. As long as you are willing to stay in the process, I will support you. You have been successful before and you will be again.
    [Patient] I hope things will be better this time. I'm willing to give it a try.

Questions to Ask Mothers

In Chapter 2, interview questions (Appendix 6) (9) are posed, followed by a guide to generate therapy recommendations. When counseling mothers who are using recreational substance(s), keep in mind that they are likely not following directions of a healthcare provider. These questions posed must be modified:

- *What is the name, strength, and dosage form of the drug?*
  Without regulation, street drugs do not have reliable strengths. Street drug guides are often composed of a multitude of pictures without labeled strengths.

- *Do you still have the prescription, or have you already filled and are taking the drug?*
  Prescription drugs have the potential to be used for recreational purpose. Avoid: if substance is not a prescription drug.

- *Why is the drug being prescribed?*
  Avoid: if substance is not a prescription drug.

- *Do you feel you need to take the drug?*
  May serve as a good start for motivational interviewing.

- *What does your physician say regarding [breastfeeding] outcomes and taking the drug?*
  Modify: what do you know about [breastfeeding] outcomes and taking the drug?

- *What is the drug dosage schedule and how often do you nurse?*
  Modify: How often do you use [the substance], and how often do you nurse?

On the other hand, these questions may not need modification.

- *How old is the baby?*
- *Was your baby full term or premature?*
- *Is your baby currently receiving any medication?*
- *Do you know how to hand express milk or do you have access to a breast pump?*
- *Is this your first [breastfed] baby?*

Summary

Healthcare providers can follow the Stepwise Approach (Appendix 6) (9) to recommend therapy modification. However, if a mother does not feel safe in the environment, she may not be honest while disclosing her substance usage history. Therefore, it is of utmost importance to implement patient-centered techniques while interviewing or counseling mothers.

Amy C. Luo

Introduction

There are many methods, including those involving drug usages, to counsel pregnant and breastfeeding women who are using or plan to use recreational and illicit drug substances. Most pharmacists, lactation consultants, nurses, and physicians are not mental healthcare professionals, psychologists, or psychiatrists. The authors are pharmacists and are not mental healthcare professionals, but we are drug experts, just as lactation consultants are lactation experts, but we, and especially we who are pharmacists, are called upon continually to counsel pregnant and breastfeeding women on drug use.

Omnibus Budget Reconciliation Act of 1990

Believe it or not, it was not until 1990 when pharmacists "officially" began to counsel patients on drug usage. Up to that time, it was only physicians who could "legally" counsel patients. The Omnibus Budget Reconciliation Act of 1990 changed all that. (10) Pharmacists by law were now required to counsel their patients on drug use. We wish to note that many pharmacists were already "unofficially" performing this crucial clinical service for their patients, many times at the dismay of the physician prescribers. An immediate consequence of the federal act was that even though only Medicaid patients were required to be counseled by pharmacists, all states eventually made this a requirement for all patients. This was to ensure that the same standard of care be provided to all patients.

To set an understanding of the standard, the following is an edited version of the Act's requirements for counseling:

While most federal laws provide the pharmacist with guidance on handling pharmaceuticals, the Omnibus Budget Reconciliation Act of 1990 (OBRA-90) placed expectations on the pharmacist on how to interact with the individual patient. While the primary goal of OBRA-90 was to save the federal government money by improving therapeutic outcomes, the method to achieve these savings was implemented by imposing on the pharmacist counseling obligations, prospective drug utilization review requirements, and record-keeping mandates.

The OBRA-90 language requires state Medicaid provider pharmacists to review Medicaid recipients' entire drug profiles before filling their prescription(s). It is intended to detect potential drug therapy problems. Computer programs can be used to assist the pharmacist in identifying potential problems. It is up to the pharmacists' professional judgment, however, as to what action to take, which could include contacting the prescriber. The following are areas for drug therapy problems that the pharmacist must screen:

- Therapeutic duplication
- Drug–disease contraindications
- Drug–drug interactions
- Incorrect drug dosage
- Incorrect duration of treatment
- Drug–allergy interactions
- Clinical abuse / misuse of medication

OBRA-90 also required states to establish standards governing patient counseling. In particular, pharmacists must offer to discuss the unique drug therapy regimen of each Medicaid recipient when filling prescriptions for them. Such discussions must include matters that are significant in the professional judgment of the pharmacist. The information that a pharmacist may discuss with a patient is found in the enumerated list below.

1. Name and description of the medication.
2. Dosage form, dosage, route of administration, and duration of drug therapy.
3. Special directions and precautions for preparation, administration, and use by the patient.

127

4. Common severe side effects, adverse effects, interactions, and therapeutic contraindications that may be encountered.

5. Techniques for self-monitoring of drug therapy.

6. Proper storage.

7. Refill information.

8. Action to be taken in the event of a missed dose.

Under OBRA-90, Medicaid pharmacy providers also must make reasonable efforts to obtain, record, and maintain certain information on Medicaid patients. This information, including pharmacist comments relevant to patient therapy, would be considered reasonable if an impartial observer could review the documentation and understand what has occurred in the past, including what the pharmacist told the patient, information discovered about the patient, and what the pharmacist thought of the patient's drug therapy. Information that would be included in documented information is listed below.

1. Name, address, and telephone number.

2. Age and gender.

3. Disease state(s) (if significant)

4. Known allergies and/or drug reactions.

5. Comprehensive list of medications and relevant devices.

6. Pharmacist's comments about the individual's drug therapy.

Summary

Clinical abuse / misuse of medication must be screened by the pharmacist as part of counseling. (11, 12) Counseling definitely includes patients who are pregnant or breastfeeding. Counseling definitely includes all drugs: the drug(s) being prescribed and all other drug substances: recreational, other prescription drugs, OTCs, herbals, supplements, controlled substance drugs, illicit drugs, drugs of abuse, and recreational drugs. Of course, pharmacists are drug experts, but lactation consultants and other healthcare professionals may also be called upon to provide counseling regarding drug use, misuse, and / or abuse. The information provided in this book is a source of background information and data to aid in the counseling process. Of course, lactation consultants and those counseling pregnant patients should consult, if necessary, with knowledgeable pharmacists as part of the medication counseling process.

Also to aid in counseling breastfeeding women, the primary author has developed Recreational Drugs Use Recommendations (Appendix 3), a benefit-risk analysis for drug usage (Appendix 4), and a Stepwise Approach to Minimizing Infant Drug Exposure (Appendix 5). (9)

Two pertinent side issues can complicate the counseling process: protection of the fetus or breastfed child and legal rights of pregnant and breastfeeding women users of illicit drugs. (13) The authors are not legal experts, but we wish to at least alert counselors of these potential issues.

The authors believe that the counseling we provide for pregnant women and breastfeeding women involves two patients: the pregnant woman and her fetus or the breastfeeding woman and her breastfed baby. Part of our society does not believe the fetus is a human being until born, and thus the fetus is not entitled to any "legal" protection. This leads to the second mitigating counseling issue: prosecution of pregnant women who use illicit drugs and drugs of abuse. All states mandate that all healthcare professionals report any knowledge of or observation of child abuse, which in many states includes reporting pregnant women to child protective services. There are those who argue that reporting of nonmedical use of controlled substances by pregnant women is "cruel and unusual punishment" for pregnant women who are considered a minority group. On the opposing side of the issue are public health concerns for the very real and significant risks to maternal, fetal, and societal wellbeing of drug use during pregnancy. The courts' reactions and rulings have been mixed.

Frank J. Nice

Chapter 11: Final Thoughts

Frank Nice; Amy C. Luo

Brianna's Story-Commitment

"It's really scary to think about the pain, and to think about not being able to make that pain go away…it's worth it for a pregnancy…it's the time between the weaning, getting the IUD taken out, and trying [that is scary]…say it takes six months!"

Brianna expressed a lot of concern about the time between complete weaning off of narcotics and the time that she got pregnant. She expressed concern that she would take one dose, would like it, feel pain reduction, and start the cycle all over again. *"That's the part that I am very scared about…and the stigma."*

The stigma of pregnancy and narcotic pain medication: *"As a patient I feel that, the doctors expect to get lied to…and they are assuming that I am going to lie to them because I am pregnant, and I am addicted. So, therefore I feel like I cannot be honest. It's like this self-fulfilling prophecy for them. Like they expect to be lied to, and I'm sure they're lied to all the time…and… there is no good answer…"*

Brianna felt significant guilt during her pregnancy about her drug use, and also was perpetually afraid that her baby would be taken away from her after birth. *"I couldn't set up a nursery, because I didn't know if I was going to bring him home… I didn't know if my baby was going to be taken away from me or not… no one would tell me anything… and all that happened was that they caught some urine for a drug test, and yes, he tested positive for narcotics, and that I needed to show you the bottle, it could be empty, but have to show the prescription bottle….and that was IT! That was it, and then I could take my baby home. And I was terrified, to the point that I couldn't' set up his nursery!"*

After taking baby home, Brianna attempted to reduce her narcotic dose, by taking just Tramadol, which she could not maintain, and then Oxycodone for breakthrough pain, but was unable to maintain that regimen either. For all of the time that her son was breastfed, she was taking at least two types of painkillers. She went back to Dilaudid and Tramadol from Oxycodone at some point during his first year of life. Both her primary care doctor and her OB assured her that breastfeeding, while taking narcotic pain medication, was fine; as well as an IBCLC from the hospital where she gave birth.

Brianna is currently still taking Dilaudid and Tramadol and occasionally muscle relaxants for the pain from her injuries. She is on a weaning dose with her primary care doctor, lowering her dose every two months.

"I felt SO guilty…." Brianna continuously expressed her desire to be a good mom, and her guilt over the fact that she was unable to quit taking narcotic painkillers during her pregnancy. She stated that she was committed to her current weaning dose so that she can have a healthy pregnancy again the second time.

Introduction

I have now been practicing as a pharmacist for almost 50 years. Professionally, I have been counseling on the use of medications during breastfeeding for the past 40 years and have published a few articles and taught a course on medication use during pregnancy. I am the father of six children and the grandfather of eight children. When I attended the University of Arizona School of Pharmacy in 1981, my initial choice for my Master's Thesis was to do a research study on the use of recreational drugs by breastfeeding mothers. I did a pilot study and was astounded by the results of this brief study. The preliminary results showed a very high use of drugs of abuse substances. Although, I chose a different topic for my research, those results have always stayed with me. The results were born out as I pursued my interest in breastfeeding and have counseled breastfeeding mothers using these drugs and have answered lactation consultants' queries about their use by breastfeeding women. It was my naive assumption back in 1979 that no woman who was breastfeeding would even think about using recreational or illicit drug substances. In reality, the situation was not so simplistic and was much more complicated than I thought.

Transitioning

Thirty-six years later in 2014, I was attending and presenting at a breastfeeding conference in Albuquerque, NM. A presentation was being offered by the Nurse-Family Partnership of Denver, CO, on helping at-risk young women. I attended because I knew one of these risks include pregnant and breastfeeding women that use recreational and illicit drugs. In fact, the first Program goal of the Nurse-Family partnership is to "improve pregnancy outcomes by helping young women engage in good preventative health practices, including.......reducing use of cigarettes, alcohol, and illegal substances." Two other goals, related to the first, are to help parents provide responsible and competent care for their children and to help parents develop a vision and plan for future pregnancies. This is especially relevant for young women with a background of poverty, conflict, and despair. The Partnership states that these women and families who partner with nurses fare better and experience less incidence of drug and alcohol abuse. I believe it is also fair to substitute lactation consultants, pharmacists, and other healthcare professionals for nurses in the Nurse-Family Partnership paradigm. I believe that many of you who have purchased this book and are now reading it have done so because of the specific belief that you can make a difference when women use drugs of abuse while pregnant and breastfeeding.

Summary

As I previously stated, the intent of this book is not to provide all inclusive counseling methods and techniques and tools, but to provide information and data that will enable you to provide objective information and counseling as it relates to the use of recreational and illicit drug substances. I believe those pregnant and breastfeeding women, in many cases, do not know exactly what these drugs are capable of doing to harm both the mother and her baby. When this information is provided in a caring, compassionate, and knowledgeable manner without value judgments and a personal agenda, we as healthcare professionals will be seen as a trusted, respected, and accessible individual. To paraphrase the Nurse-Family Partnership: It is about changing lives for our generation of mothers and fathers and children and all future generations of our and their descendants.

Frank J. Nice, Father and Pharmacist

Introduction

When I register for the American Pharmacists Association (APhA) conferences, anyone who has practiced pharmacy for five years or less is labeled as a "New Practitioner." As a New Practitioner, I have been fortunate to serve as a pharmacist for the Navajo Nation with the Indian Health Service (IHS).

IHS is known for having developed the method of counseling taught at pharmacy schools across the nation and is the basis of the APhA counseling competition. The IHS method of counseling asks three open-ended questions:

1. What did your doctor* tell you about this medication (a question about purpose of medication use)?
2. How did your doctor* tell you to take this medication (a question about directions)?
3. What did your doctor* tell you to expect from this medication (a question about side effects)?

Experimenting with the abbreviated way of counseling versus applying the developed method of counseling revealed the apparent improvement of the counseling conversation. The IHS method encouraged an open line of communication between the pharmacist and the patient. Patients are much more comfortable when I introduce myself by stating my name, my role, the purpose of counseling, and state that their questions will be kept private. Patients listen attentively when I ask them open-ended questions, as opposed to yes or no questions. Patients demonstrate their understanding better when they reiterate the directions given. Patients ask relevant, and sometimes personal questions, when they believe that their questions will be kept private, and that the pharmacist has the knowledge to help his or her particular case.

Transitioning

I share my experience, stories, and tips with pharmacy students on rotation. They tell me stories of patients extending a handshake because they are so grateful, patients admitting to noncompliance, and patients revealing their concerns never brought up to their doctors*.

Over the past four years, I did not encounter mothers who spoke openly about their experiences breastfeeding while considering the consequences of recreational drug use. However, with my experience with patients asking very private questions and the feedback from my pharmacy students, makes me believe that when a breastfeeding mother uses recreational drugs, she may feel comfortable enough to ask openly, or at least allude to her concerns in the counseling room.

When Dr. Frank J. Nice approached me to collaborate on this book with him, I said "yes" right away. However, as soon as I started writing, I realized that I had no real life experience to offer. Instead, I learned so much from writing this book. Quora.com is a question-and-answer website where questions are asked, answered, edited, and organized by its community of users. When I asked on Quora, "What is it like to use marijuana and breastfeed at the same time?," the only comment I received was, "Is this a real question?" Case reports of recreational drug use are cited in lactation resources. Dr. Nice's contacts also graciously offered stories from their practices. I learned that recreational drug use during breastfeeding is a real concern.

Summary

Towards the end of writing this book, I met Scott Carroll, MD, a child psychiatrist who happened to sit in the same row with me on a plane. Dr. Carroll shared this from his practice: Some patients whose behaviors indicate that they are on a recreational substance may present with a clean drug screen. Synthetics that do not show up in drug screens are not discussed in this book, as there is little information available currently. There is also a variety of information not covered. The intent of "Recreational Drugs and Drugs Used to Treat Addicted Mothers: Impact on Pregnancy and Breastfeeding" is not to provide a comprehensive list of substances, but to bring awareness to this topic, to serve as an aid in making clinical decisions, and to provide tips when addressing patients with this issue.

*Doctors as in a generalized term for doctors, nurse practitioners, physician assistants, any healthcare providers who prescribe medication for the patients.

Amy C. Luo, Pharmacist

Appendices

Appendix 1: Controlled Drug Substances Schedules

Appendix 2: Marijuana

Appendix 3: Recreational Drugs Use Recommendations for Breastfeeding

Appendix 4: Benefits of Breastfeeding and Risks of Not Breastfeeding

Appendix 5: Questions to Ask in Breastfeeding / Medication Situations

Appendix 6: Stepwise Approach to Minimizing Infant Drug Exposure While Breastfeeding

Appendix 1: Controlled Drug Substances Schedules

The Controlled Substances Act (CSA) Title II of the Comprehensive Drug Abuse Prevention and Control Act of 1970 is the federal U.S. drug policy under which the manufacture, importation, possession, use and distribution of certain narcotics, stimulants, depressants, hallucinogens, anabolic steroids and other chemicals are regulated. (1) The CSA was signed into law by President Richard Nixon on October 27, 1970. The addition, deletion or change of schedule of a medicine or substance may be requested by the U.S. Drug Enforcement Agency (DEA), the Department of Health and Human Services, the U.S. Food and Drug Administration (FDA), or from any other party via petition to the DEA.

The DEA implements the CSA and may prosecute violators of these laws at both the domestic and international level. Within the CSA there are five schedules (I-V) that are used to classify drugs based upon their abuse potential, medical applications, and safety. Individuals who order, handle, store, and distribute controlled substances must be registered with the DEA to perform these functions. They must maintain accurate inventories, records and security of the controlled substances.

The abuse rate is a determinate factor in the scheduling of the drug; for example, Schedule I drugs are considered the most dangerous class of drugs with a high potential for abuse and potentially severe psychological and/or physical dependence. As the drug schedule changes-- Schedule II, Schedule III, etc., so does the abuse potential-- Schedule V drugs represents the least potential for abuse. Both the basic or parent chemical and the salts, isomers, and salts of isomers, esters, ethers and derivatives may also be classified as controlled substances.

Note that a substance need not be listed as a controlled substance to be treated as a Schedule I substance for criminal prosecution. A controlled substance analogue is a substance which is intended for human consumption and is structurally or pharmacologically substantially similar to or is represented as being similar to a Schedule I or Schedule II substance and is not an approved medication in the United States. (See 21 U.S.C. §802(32)(A) for the definition of a controlled substance analogue and 21 U.S.C. §813 for the schedule.)

Schedule I

Schedule I drugs, substances, or chemicals are defined as drugs with no currently accepted medical use and a high potential for abuse. Schedule I drugs are the most dangerous drugs of all the drug schedules with potentially severe psychological or physical dependence. Some examples of Schedule I drugs are:

> Heroin, lysergic acid diethylamide (LSD), marijuana (cannabis), 3,4-methylenedioxymethamphetamine (ecstasy), methaqualone, and peyote

NOTE: Tetrahydrocannabinol (THC, marijuana) is still considered a Schedule 1 drug by the DEA, even though some U.S. states have legalized marijuana for personal, recreational, or medical use.

Schedule II

Schedule II drugs, substances, or chemicals are defined as drugs with a high potential for abuse, less abuse potential than Schedule I drugs, with use potentially leading to severe psychological or physical dependence. These drugs are also considered dangerous. Some examples of Schedule II drugs are:

> Combination products with less than 15 milligrams of hydrocodone per dosage unit (Vicodin),cocaine, methamphetamine, methadone, hydromorphone (Dilaudid), meperidine (Demerol), oxycodone (OxyContin), fentanyl, Dexedrine, Adderall, and Ritalin

Schedule III

Schedule III drugs, substances, or chemicals are defined as drugs with a moderate to low potential for physical and psychological dependence. Schedule III drug abuse potential is less than Schedule I and Schedule II drugs but more than Schedule IV. Some examples of Schedule III drugs are:

> Products containing less than 90 milligrams of codeine per dosage unit (Tylenol with codeine), ketamine, anabolic steroids, testosterone

Schedule IV

Schedule IV drugs, substances, or chemicals are defined as drugs with a low potential for abuse and low risk of dependence. Some examples of Schedule IV drugs are:

> Xanax, Soma, Valium, Ativan, Talwin, Ambien, Tramadol

Schedule V

Schedule V drugs, substances, or chemicals are defined as drugs with lower potential for abuse than Schedule IV and consist of preparations containing limited quantities of certain narcotics. Schedule V drugs are generally used for antidiarrheal, antitussive, and analgesic purposes. Some examples of Schedule V drugs are:

> Cough preparations with less than 200 milligrams of codeine or per 100 milliliters: Robitussin AC, Lomotil, Motofen, Lyrica, Parepectolin

Appendix 2: Marijuana

Botanical name: *Cannabis sativa*

Other common names: weed, pot, herb, bud, dope, spliff, reefer, grass, ganja, 420, chronic, MJ, Mary Jane, gangster, boom, skunk. There are over 200 street names for marijuana.

What is Marijuana?

Marijuana is a green, brown or gray mixture of dried, shredded leaves, stems, seeds and flowers of the hemp plant *Cannabis sativa*. (1) Marijuana is used as a psychoactive (i.e., mind altering) recreational drug, for certain medical ailments, and for religious and spiritual purposes. Sinsemilla, hash/hashish (resinous form) and hash oil (sticky black liquid) are stronger forms of marijuana.

How Does Marijuana Work?

The main active chemical in marijuana is THC (delta-9-tetrahydrocannabinol). It is a psychoactive ingredient. The highest concentrations of THC are found in the leaves and flowers. When marijuana smoke is inhaled, THC rapidly passes from the lungs into the bloodstream and is carried to the brain and other organs throughout the body. THC from the marijuana acts on specific receptors in the brain, called cannabinoid receptors, starting a chain of cellular reactions that finally lead to the euphoria, or "high," that users experience.

Certain areas in the brain, such as the hippocampus, the cerebellum, the basal ganglia, and the cerebral cortex, have a higher concentration of cannabinoid receptors. These areas influence memory, concentration, pleasure, coordination, sensory, and time perception. Therefore these functions are most adversely affected by marijuana use.

Marijuana's strength is correlated to the amount of THC it contains and the effects on the user depend on the strength or potency of THC. The THC content in marijuana has been increasing since the 1970s. For the year 2007, estimates from confiscated marijuana indicate that it contains almost 10 percent THC on average. There are many other chemicals found in marijuana, many of which may adversely affect health. Marijuana contains over 60 different cannabinoid compounds related to THC, including cannabidiol, cannabinol, and β-caryophyllene.

Marijuana is usually smoked as a cigarette (called a joint or a nail) or in a pipe or bong. In recent years, it has appeared in blunts, which are cigars that have been emptied of tobacco and refilled with marijuana, often in combination with another drug, such as crack. The "blunts" retain tobacco leaf used to wrap the cigar and therefore it combines marijuana's active ingredients with nicotine and other harmful chemicals. Some users also mix marijuana into food or use it to brew tea.

Medicinal Use of THC

In the United States, the Controlled Substances Act (CSA) of 1990 classifies marijuana as a Schedule I substance, which has no approved medical use and has high potential for abuse. (2, 3) However, some US states have legalized the use of marijuana for medical or recreational use. Prescription medicines containing synthetic cannabinoids (THC) are already available.

- Marinol (dronabinol) - Classified as Schedule III

- Cesamet (nabilone) - Classified as Schedule II

Both medications are used to treat chemotherapy patients who have nausea, vomiting, and loss of appetite. However, Marinol is also approved to treat HIV patients with cachexia (weight loss, muscle atrophy, fatigue, and loss of appetite).

Studies have also been done which show that THC and cannabidiol (CBD) provide therapeutic benefit for Multiple Sclerosis (MS) spasticity symptoms. In Canada, Europe, the UK, Spain, Germany, Denmark, the Czech Republic, Sweden, and New Zealand, Sativex, an oral sublingual spray, is available for adjunctive use in MS neuropathic pain and cancer-related pain. Sativex® is composed of plant-derived extracts of THC and cannabidiol, not synthetic cannabinoids. In 2013, Sativex® was in Phase II and III clinical trials for US approval for use in MS spasticity and cancer pain, and has the adopted generic name of nabiximols. Dronabinol has also been used in Europe for treatment of MS-related pain.

Marijuana has also been used for glaucoma to lower intraocular pressure (IOP), but research does not show that marijuana has a better effect than currently approved glaucoma medications. Studies have shown that smoked, oral, or IV use may have an effect on lowering IOP, but topically applied marijuana derivatives to the eye did not have an effect. Marijuana is not FDA approved for use in glaucoma and may lead to other side effects, such as increased heart rate and lowered blood pressure. However, in some US states, marijuana is used for glaucoma under medical marijuana programs.

Extent of Marijuana Use

In January 2014, marijuana was noted by the National Institute on Drug Abuse as being the most widely used illicit drug in the US. (1) Globally, between 129 and 191 million people aged 15 to 64 used marijuana at least one time in 2008, or 2.9 to 3.4% of the world's population. In North America, 29.5 million people used marijuana at least once in 2008. According to the 2010 National Survey on Drug Use and Health (NSDUH), marijuana was used by 76.8% of current illicit drug users (defined as having used the drug at some time in the 30 days before the survey) and was the only drug used by 60.1% of them.

Data indicate that in 2008 marijuana was responsible for about 17% (322,000) of all admissions to treatment facilities in the United States. Only opiates have a higher admission rate among abused substances. Marijuana admissions were primarily male (74%), white (49%), and young (30% were in the 12-17 age range). Starting marijuana by age 14 was a common factor among 56% of those admitted for treatment.

According to the 2011 *National Survey on Drug Use and Health*, 2.6 million Americans aged 12 or older used marijuana for the first time in the 12 months prior to being surveyed (roughly 7,200 new users per day), which is similar to the 2009-2010 rate (2.4 million each), but higher than the estimates in 2002 through 2008. (1) Close to 58% of the 2.4 million recent marijuana users were younger than age 18 when they first used. Among all youths aged 12 to 17, an estimated 5.5% had used marijuana for the first time within the past year, which was similar to the rate in 2010 (5.2%).

The 2012 Monitoring the Future survey indicates that marijuana use among 8th-, 10th-, and 12th-graders, which had shown a consistent rise over 2010 and 2011, leveled off in 2012. Daily marijuana use increased significantly in all three grades in 2010, 1.2%, 3.3. %, and 6.1% in grades 8, 10 and 12, which computes to roughly one out of every 16 high school seniors who smoke marijuana daily. (1) These trends increased slightly in the higher grades in 2012, with 1.1%, 3.5%, and 6.5% in grades 8, 10, and 12 using marijuana daily.

Perceived risk and individual disapproval of marijuana is a leading indicator of marijuana use among teens in the U.S. In all grades in 2012, those who perceived smoking marijuana as harmful and the proportion who disapprove of the drug's use have slightly declined, suggesting use may increase in upcoming years. In 2012, 37% of 8th graders, 69% of 10th graders, and 82% of 12th graders reported marijuana as being fairly or very easy to get. It thus seems clear that marijuana has remained highly accessible to the older teens.

Effects During Pregnancy and Breastfeeding

Any drug of abuse can affect a mother's health. THC can cross the placenta, so there is potential for problems in the fetus. (1) THC can depress fetal heart rates and change fetal brain wave electrical patterns. Studies have found that babies born to mothers who used marijuana during pregnancy were smaller than those born to mothers who did not use the drug. In general, smaller babies are more likely to develop health problems. Tests given to children at 48 months of age whose mothers used marijuana during pregnancy have shown lower verbal and memory scores compared to children whose mother did not use marijuana. Babies born to adolescents who used marijuana during pregnancy have also shown adverse effects on the neurological behavior of the newborns in the first 24 to 78 hours after delivery.

A nursing mother who uses marijuana passes some of the THC to the baby in her breast milk. Research indicates that use by a mother during the first month of breastfeeding can impair the infant's motor development. Pregnant and nursing women should avoid marijuana use.

Marijuana Side Effects (1)

What are the short-term side effects of Marijuana use? Side effects of marijuana use will be variable from person to person, depending upon strength and amount of marijuana used and if the user is occasionally or chronically exposed to THC. (1) The short-term effects of marijuana use include problems with memory and learning; distorted perception (sights, sounds, time, and touch); difficulty in thinking and problem solving; loss of coordination and motor skills; and increased heart rate, anxiety, bloodshot eyes, and dry mouth. Reaction time may be impaired while driving. Panic attacks, paranoia, and psychosis may occur acutely and be more common in psychiatric patients. For chronic users, the impact on memory and learning can last for days or weeks after its acute effects wear off. Marijuana may be cut on the street with more dangerous substances that may lead to more serious side effects.

THC in marijuana is strongly absorbed by fatty tissues in various organs. Generally, traces of THC can be detected by standard urine testing methods several days after a smoking session. In heavy chronic users, traces can sometimes be detected for weeks after they have stopped using marijuana.

What are the long-term side effects of Marijuana use? People who smoke marijuana often have the same respiratory problems as cigarette smokers. These individuals may have daily cough and phlegm, symptoms of chronic bronchitis, and more frequent chest colds. They are also at greater risk of getting lung infections like pneumonia. Marijuana contains some of the same, and sometimes even more, of the cancer-causing chemicals found in cigarette smoke. A study from 2009 suggests that regular and long-term use of marijuana may increase the risk for testicular cancer.

When people smoke marijuana for years they can suffer negative consequences. For example, because marijuana affects brain function, the ability to do complex tasks could be compromised, as well as the pursuit of academic, athletic, or other life goals that require you to be 100% focused and alert. Long-term abuse of marijuana may lead to addiction.

Marijuana also may affect mental health. Studies show that early use may increase the risk of developing psychosis (a severe mental disorder in which there is a loss of contact with reality), including false ideas about what is happening (delusions) and seeing or hearing things that aren't there (hallucinations), particularly if you carry a genetic vulnerability to the disease. Also, rates of marijuana use are often higher in people with symptoms of depression or anxiety.

Effects of Marijuana on Other Organs (1)

Effects on the Heart

Shortly after smoking marijuana the heart rate increases drastically and may remain elevated for up to three hours. This effect may be enhanced if other drugs are taken with marijuana. One study has suggested that the risk of heart attack may increase by up to 4.8-fold in the first hour after smoking marijuana. The effect may be due to the increased heart rate, as well as altered heart rhythms. The risk of heart attack may be greater in those with specific risk factors, such as patients with high blood pressure, heart arrhythmia, or other cardiac disease.

Effects on the Lungs

After smoking marijuana, the bronchial passage relaxes and becomes enlarged, and the blood vessels in the eyes expand, making the eyes look red. Studies have shown that marijuana is an irritant to the lungs. Marijuana users tend to inhale more deeply and hold their breath longer than tobacco smokers do, which further increase the lungs' exposure to carcinogenic smoke. Marijuana smokers can have many of the same respiratory problems as tobacco smokers, such as daily cough and phlegm production, more frequent acute chest illness, and a heightened risk of lung infections. A case-controlled study from 2006 found no links between marijuana use and lung cancer, but no evidence-based consensus has been definitively made on the absolute risk of lung cancer with marijuana use.

Effects of Heavy Marijuana Use on Social Behavior (1)

Heavy marijuana abusers may show low achievement in important life measures, including mental and physical health, and career. Marijuana affects memory, judgment, and perception. Learning and attention skills are impaired among people who use it heavily. Longitudinal research on marijuana use among young people below college age indicates those who use marijuana have lower achievement than non-users, more acceptance of deviant behavior, more delinquent behavior and aggression, greater rebelliousness, poorer relationships with parents, and more associations with delinquent and drug-using friends.

Smoking marijuana can make driving dangerous. The cerebellum is the section of our brain that controls balance and coordination. When THC affects the cerebellum's function, it can cause disaster on the road. Research shows that drivers have slower reaction times, impaired judgment, and problems responding to signals and sounds if driving while under the influence of THC.

Addictive Potential (1)

A drug is addicting if it causes compulsive, uncontrollable drug craving, seeking, and use, even in the face of negative health and social consequences. Research suggests that roughly 9% of users become addicted to marijuana, with higher rates if the user starts at a young age (17%) and in those who use marijuana daily (25-50%). While not everyone who uses marijuana becomes addicted, when a user begins to seek out and take the drug compulsively, that person is said to be dependent or addicted to the drug.

Long-term users who try to quit can experience withdrawal symptoms, such as sleeplessness, irritability, anxiety, decreased appetite, and drug craving. Withdrawal symptoms usually begin about a day after the person stops using marijuana, peaks in two to three days, and may take one to two weeks to subside.

Some heavy users develop a tolerance to marijuana, meaning the user needs larger doses to get the same desired results that he or she used to get from smaller amounts.

Medical Marijuana (1)

As of July 2014, 23 states and the District of Columbia legally allow marijuana for personal medical use. Rules surrounding the use of medical marijuana vary by state. The first state in the union to legalize the medical use of marijuana was California in 1996. Other states that allow medical marijuana include: Alaska, Arizona, California, Colorado, Connecticut,

Delaware, Hawaii, Illinois, Maine, Maryland, Massachusetts, Michigan, Minnesota, Montana, Nevada, New Hampshire, New Jersey, New Mexico, New York, Oregon, Rhode Island, Vermont, Washington, and the District of Columbia. It is important to recognize that these state marijuana laws do not change the fact that using marijuana continues to be an offense under Federal law.

Medical marijuana in the US is controlled at the state level. Per federal law, cannabis is illegal as noted in the Controlled Substances Act (3), but the federal government has stated they will not actively prosecute patients and caregivers complying with state medical marijuana laws. However, use of medical marijuana outside of the state laws for illegal use or trafficking will not be tolerated by state or federal governments.

There are eight medical conditions for which patients can use cannabis:

- Cancer
- Glaucoma
- HIV/AIDS
- Muscle spasms
- Seizures
- Severe pain
- Severe nausea
- Cachexia or dramatic weight loss and muscle atrophy (wasting syndrome)

According to various state laws, medical marijuana can be used for treatment of other debilitating medical conditions, such as decompensated cirrhosis, amyotrophic lateral sclerosis, Alzheimer's disease, and post-traumatic stress disorder. Not all states that approve medical marijuana have enacted laws to allow its use for all of these conditions. Another difference between states - the amount of marijuana for medical use that can be possessed by the individual patient or primary caregiver varies, but may include dried marijuana and live plants.

In healthcare, the use of marijuana for medical reasons is controversial. In November 2013, the American Medical Association (AMA) voted to retain an official position that "cannabis is a dangerous drug and as such is a public health concern," but also acknowledged the changing attitudes toward marijuana among the American public. The AMA calls for laws "to emphasize public-health-based strategies to address and reduce cannabis use" and state that criminal laws for the illegal possession of marijuana for personal recreational use focus on "public health based strategies, rather than incarceration."

The American Medical Association (AMA) encourages continued research of marijuana and related cannabinoids in patients who have serious conditions. AMA also states that marijuana's status as a federal schedule I controlled substance should be reviewed "with the goal of facilitating the conduct of clinical research and development of cannabinoid-based medicines, and alternate delivery methods. This should not be viewed as an endorsement of state-based medical cannabis programs, the legalization of marijuana, or that scientific evidence on the therapeutic use of cannabis meets the current standards for a prescription drug product." The AMA continues to stand strong against the legalization of marijuana for recreational use. The AMA also rejected a proposal to advocate for the "sale of cannabis to be regulated on a state-based level."

Several states are now considering or have passed bills to allow legalization of medical marijuana oil (CBD Oil or Realm Oil) for intractable seizures in children with Dravet Syndrome. These children can suffer 40 more seizures per day; the seizures are often prolonged in length. The oil is made from a special strain of marijuana called "Charlotte's Web" that has extremely low levels of tetrahydrocannabinol (THC), the psychoactive ingredient in marijuana that leads to the "high." However, the strain has elevated levels of cannabidiol, or CBD, a non-psychoactive component that has been shown to have a number of therapeutic benefits, including those that limit seizure activity. The oil is taken in an oral liquid form, not smoked like traditional marijuana. News media have showcased several families from states that do not allow the CBD Oil. These families have moved to Colorado from their home states to access the oil legally for their children who suffer from the debilitating seizures. Legislation is currently under review in several states to allow the oil for children with this debilitating seizure condition. As of June 7, 2015, in addition to the states that allow medical marijuana, 15 states had okayed the use of CBD Oil: these states include Utah, Texas, Alabama, Kentucky, Missouri, Wisconsin, Mississippi, Tennessee, Georgia, South Carolina, Iowa, Florida, North Carolina, Virginia, and Illinois.

Political leaders, US government officials, healthcare providers and medical organizations take differing views of the benefits and risks of medical marijuana. Proponents state that marijuana has valid medical uses and further research should be pursued, while opponents list concerns about health risks, and the "gateway" effect of marijuana that can lead to more dangerous drug abuse, among other issues. Nonetheless, legalization of medical marijuana continues to be pursued at the state level, with pending legislation in multiple states.

Recreational Use of Marijuana (1)

In 2012, voters in Colorado and Washington states passed initiatives legalizing marijuana for adults 21 and older under state law. The states of Oregon and Alaska, as well as Washington, D.C., also voted to approve recreational use of marijuana in November 2014. It is important to note that the federal government still considers marijuana a dangerous drug and that the illegal distribution and sale of marijuana is a serious crime. Under the Controlled Substances Act (CSA), marijuana is still considered a Schedule 1 drug. Cultivation and distribution of marijuana are felonies; possession for personal use is a misdemeanor; possession of "paraphernalia" is also illegal. Cultivating 100 plants or more carries a mandatory minimum sentence of five years according to federal statutes.

That being said, it is unlikely that the federal government is interested in pursuing individuals complying with state-mandated regulations surrounding legalized marijuana for recreational use, although the CSA law still gives them authority to do so.

The Department of Justice (DOJ) has attempted to clarify this issue. On August 29, 2013, the DOJ issued guidance to Federal prosecutors concerning marijuana enforcement under the CSA. The DOJ is focused on priorities, such as:

- Preventing the distribution to minors.
- Preventing revenues from sale of marijuana towards criminal activity.
- Preventing diversion of marijuana from states where it is legal to states where it is not legal.
- Preventing state-legalized marijuana from being a cover for other illegal drugs or activity.
- Prevent violence and guns in the cultivation and distribution of marijuana.
- Prevent drugged driving and other public health issues.
- Prevent the use of public land for marijuana cultivation.
- Preventing marijuana possession or use on federal property.

Additional states may undertake or pursue citizen petitions in the future to legalize the recreational use of marijuana. According to the Brookings Institute, Presidential years bring out an electorate more favorable to marijuana legalization than the off-year electorate. Other states pursuing legalization may include California, Arizona, Nevada, Massachusetts, Montana, Rhode Island, and Vermont. Maine and Michigan citizen voters have also passed legalization of marijuana for recreational use, but state law will likely override these voter referendums; only medical marijuana is currently legal according to state law in these states.

A majority of Americans support legalization of marijuana–52% pro versus 45% con–according to findings from a Pew Research Center survey in March 2013. Support for marijuana legalization has increased dramatically since 2010, by 11 percentage points.

Colorado

Colorado passed Colorado Amendment 64 on November 6, 2012, allowing the sale and possession of recreational marijuana. (4) Adults 21 years and older can grow up to three immature and three flowering, mature cannabis plants privately and in a locked space. Adults can legally possess all the cannabis from the plants in the place it was grown, but when traveling away from this place may only possess one ounce in total. In addition, an adult may give up to one ounce to another adult at least 21 years of age; it cannot be sold.

On January 1, 2014, retail marijuana shops opened for business in Colorado, and sales of marijuana are now taxed at the state level. Retail taxes on recreational marijuana can be lofty; in the Denver metro area, they can exceed 20%. In January 2014 alone, Colorado pulled in over $2 million in taxes from recreational marijuana sales.

Specific city and county laws have been enacted to regulate how citizens and tourists may possess and consume marijuana. Penalties exist for driving while under the influence of marijuana. Someone driving under the influence of marijuana is considered impaired when five nanograms per milliliter (ng/mL) of blood or more of active THC is detected, according to the Colorado Department of Transportation. Tourists to the city may purchase a quarter ounce at retail shops, instead of the one ounce for state residents. The newly formed Colorado Marijuana Enforcement Division of the Department of Revenue regulates recreational marijuana in the state.

Washington

On November 6, 2013, the state of Washington passed Washington Initiative 502, also legalizing marijuana possession and sale for recreational use for adults 21 years and older. (5) The initiative was approved by popular vote, passing by roughly 56 to 44%. Like Colorado, Washington taxes marijuana cultivation and sales. Washington's retail tax rate on marijuana is somewhat higher than Colorado's, at roughly 30 to 40%. However, additional excise taxes are implemented in the supply chain. It has been reported that tax dollars will be directed to schools, youth drug abuse programs, and campaigns to hinder driving while under the influence of marijuana.

Washington residents cannot grow recreational marijuana for personal use, although they can cultivate medical marijuana if it is approved by a physician for their use. Residents may possess up to one ounce of marijuana, previously a misdemeanor charge. The same rules for driving under the influence in Colorado apply to Washington residents. The commercial market in Washington State is regulated by the Washington State Liquor Control Board.

Washington Senate Bill 5052 was signed during April 2015 (5). The law provides for new patient possession limits, new patient grow limits, new sales tax requirements, new collective garden rules, and new licensing guidelines. The major change is that previous marijuana dispensaries will be absorbed from the Liquor Control Board to this state's highly regulated recreational cannabis market, dubbed the Liquor and Cannabis Control Board.

Appendix 3: Recreational Drug Use Recommendations for Breastfeeding

After many years of breastfeeding consultation and communication with Lactation Consultants, the primary author developed these **recommendations** for healthcare professionals and breastfeeding mothers: (1)

- If recreational drugs have been used, interrupt breastfeeding for 24-48 hours after the last dose.

- Babies may test positive for drug for days to weeks.

- Extreme warnings: cocaine, LSD, phencyclidine (angel dust, PCP), hallucinogenic drugs, amphetamines, IV heroin.

- PCP and cocaine may be the most dangerous of all drugs because these substances may remain in the baby's system for weeks after the last maternal dose (they have long half-life metabolites).

- Social considerations include how heavy a substance user the mother is, as well as her ability to care for her baby while under the influence.

- There is a need to assess the dependability of the mother.

- Discontinuing breastfeeding should be recommended for high-risk mothers.

- For low-risk mothers, explain drug transfer into breast milk and the hazards of the drug substance to the baby.

- Explain hazards of Hepatitis B and HIV transfer in unprotected babies should the mother become infected.

- Explain that the baby possibly could be drug-screen positive for LONG periods.

- Explain the legal consequences of drug-screen tests in babies, even if the drug substance is "legal" or "medically" necessary.

- Healthcare professionals should recognize the importance of breastfeeding: use the recommended benefits/risk analysis.

- Healthcare professionals should recognize that some drugs of abuse are largely only dangerous for brief intervals following use.

- Healthcare professionals should counsel mothers strongly and recommend that the mother be re-screened several weeks to one month post-partum.

- If the mother tests positive for heroin, cocaine, amphetamines, or hallucinogens, she should stop breastfeeding.

- Screen the baby.

Most questions healthcare professionals hear are usually about **alcohol** use:

- Alcohol rapidly exchanges between plasma and breast milk.

- One study has shown that mothers' alcohol resulted in a 23% reduction in the amount of milk ingested by babies, which may be due to the taste of alcohol in the breast milk.

- Prolactin production may be inhibited by alcohol, but is definitely not known.

- Maternal alcohol blood levels have to reach 300 mg% before significant side effects affect the baby.

- Breastfeeding can be resumed after moderate alcohol use as soon as the mother feels normal.

- Recommend interrupting breastfeeding for one (1) hour per drink or until the mother is sober.

Marijuana use is now "legal" in many states, but:

- The long-term effects of marijuana on breastfed infants are not entirely known.

- Experts advise that mothers who use marijuana must stop breastfeeding or ask for medical assistance to stop its use, in order for the mother to provide her baby with all the benefits of human milk.

- Some mothers who smoke marijuana away from the baby do not realize the THC from the marijuana is concentrated in breast milk and is absorbed by the nursing babies.

- When mothers are informed of that fact, they may be more willing to give up marijuana for the benefit of their babies.

In conclusion, from both philosophical and scientific viewpoints, recreational drugs of abuse should be contraindicated during breastfeeding as they are hazardous, not only to the nursling, but to the mother as well.

Appendix 4: Benefits of Breastfeeding and Risks of Not Breastfeeding

Benefits of Breastfeeding and Risks of Not Breastfeeding (1)

Benefits of Breastfeeding	Risks of Not Breastfeeding
<ul><li>Bonding between mother and child</li><li>Better recovery with less blood loss at birth</li><li>Delays return of a woman's ovulation and menstruation for a variable 20 to 30 weeks or more, providing a natural means of child spacing for many.</li><li>Enhances feelings of attachment between mother and baby</li></ul> Infants receive: <ul><li>Immunoglobulin</li><li>Enhanced immune response to inoculations against:<ul><li>Polio</li><li>Tetanus</li></ul></li></ul>	Mothers will have increased risks of: <ul><li>Post-partum hemorrhage by increasing level of oxytocin, which stimulates uterine contractions</li><li>Pre-menopausal breast cancer</li><li>Ovarian cancer</li><li>Heart disease</li><li>Osteoporosis</li><li>Anemia</li><li>Obesity</li><li>Type 2 diabetes for women without a history of gestational diabetes</li></ul> Infants will have increased risks of: <ul><li>SIDS (Sudden Infant Death Syndrome)</li><li>Infectious Diseases</li><li>Diarrhea</li><li>Ear Infections</li><li>Upper Respiratory Tract Infections</li><li>Meningitis</li><li>Bowel Diseases<ul><li>Chron's Disease</li></ul></li></ul>

- Diphtheria
- Influenza
- Nutrients
- Growth factors
- Lipoproteins/cholesterol needed for brain and nerve development

In the adolescent and adult lives of infants, associations with:

- Lower mean blood pressure
- Lower total serum cholesterol
- Lower prevalence of type 2 diabetes

- Ulcerative Colitis
- Cancer
  - Hodgkin's Disease
  - Leukemia
- Diabetes
- Obesity
- Asthma
- Eczema
- Cavities
- Decreased IQ (by 8-15 points)
- Acute infections
  - Diarrhea
  - Pneumonia
  - Ear infection
  - *Haemonphilus influenza*
  - Meningitis
  - Urinary tract infection
- Chronic conditions in the future
  - Type I diabetes
  - Ulcerative colitis
  - Crohn's disease

Appendix 5: Questions to Ask in Breastfeeding/Medication Situations

1. What is the name, strength, and dosage form of the drug?

This is the basic information needed to evaluate any situation involving drug use.

2. Do you still have the prescription? Or, have you already filled it and are taking the drug?

Asking this question helps get the proper perspective as to the stage of the drug / breastfeeding situation that is being evaluated. The mother may be seeking advice on whether to continue breastfeeding, if and when she takes the drug. She may be questioning whether she is acting correctly by taking the drug and continuing to breastfeed. And she may have concerns about possible adverse effects on her infant.

3. Why is the drug being prescribed?

Knowing the answer to this question can help the mother determine if, in fact, the drug is really necessary in a particular situation. This is best decided with the prescribing physician.

4. Do you feel you need to take the drug?

If the drug is being prescribed for a relatively benign condition, the mother may be willing to endure some personal inconvenience to spare the infant from potential effects of the drug. This is also best decided in conjunction with the prescribing physician.

5. What does your doctor say regarding breastfeeding outcome and taking the drug?

A doctor's philosophy about breastfeeding and knowledge of drug effects on breastfeeding can play a large role in the doctor's opinion as to whether the mother should continue to breastfeed. With knowledge of the doctor's philosophy in relation to her own views on breastfeeding, the mother can decide if she wants to further pursue the physician's decision. If a physician's and a mother's philosophies are in conflict, the mother should seek a second opinion.

6. What is the drug dosage schedule and how often do you nurse?

If a drug must be taken by a mother, and she wishes to continue to breastfeed, it may be possible to schedule the doses so that peak plasma and milk levels of the drug do not coincide with breastfeeding sessions. In most cases, it's best for the mother to breastfeed just before taking a dose of a drug and / or at least two hours after taking a dose. Short-acting drugs taken on an every three to six hour schedule usually reach peak plasma and milk levels in approximately one hour.

7. How old is the baby?

Knowing this gives an indication of the infant's ability to handle a particular drug. Also it aids determining the infant's feeding schedule which may influence dosage scheduling.

8. Was your baby full-term or premature?

The answer to this question supplies added information that helps determine the infant's ability to detoxify drugs.

9. What is your baby's weight?

This fact may be relevant to the quantity of the drug the baby may be able to tolerate without any adverse effects.

10. Is your baby currently receiving any medication?

Any medication that the infant is receiving can interact with medication the infant receives through breast milk.

11. Do you know how to hand-express milk or do you have access to a breast pump?

In some cases, breastfeeding can be stopped temporarily while a drug is administered. In these situations, the mother must hand-express milk or pump her breast to prevent breast engorgement and to maintain her milk supply. The mother can learn to hand-express milk or to use a breast pump, if necessary, from lactation consultants or La Leche League consultants.

12. Is this your first breastfed baby?

Mothers who have breastfed in the past will be more knowledgeable about the whole breastfeeding process. A mother who is breastfeeding for the first time may find it more difficult to come to a decision regarding the use of a drug. Involving a breastfeeding consultant in the process, if this is acceptable to the mother, may be useful.

Appendix 6: Stepwise Approach to Minimizing Infant Drug Exposure While Breastfeeding

1. **Withhold the Drug:** Avoid the use of non-essential medications by enlisting the mother's cooperation.

2. **Try Non-Drug Therapies:** Suggested therapies include:
   - Analgesics: relaxation techniques, massage, warm baths. Cough, cold, allergy products: saline nose drops, cool mist, steam.
   - Anti-asthmatics: avoid known allergens, particularly animals.
   - Antacids: eat small meals, sleep with head propped, avoid head-bending activities, and avoid gas-forming foods.
   - Laxatives: eat high fiber cereal, prunes, or hot liquids with breakfast
   - Anti-diarrheals: discontinue solids for 12-24 hours, increase fluids, and eat toast / saltine crackers.

3. **Delay Therapy:** Mothers who are ready to wean the infant might be able to delay elective drug therapy or elective surgery.

4. **Choose Drugs That Pass Poorly Into Milk:** Within some drug classes, there are large differences among class members in drug distribution into milk.

5. **Choose More Breastfeeding Compatible Dosage Forms:** Take lowest recommended dose, avoid extra-strength and long acting preparations, avoid combination ingredient products.

6. **Choose an Alternative Route of Administration:** Local application of drugs to the affected maternal site may minimize drug concentrations in milk and subsequently the infant's dose.

7. **Avoid Nursing at Times of Peak Drug Concentrations in Milk:** Nursing before a dose is given may avoid the peak drug concentrations in milk that occur about one to three hours after an oral dose. This works best for drugs with short half-lives.

8. **Administer the Drug Before the Infant's Longest Sleep Period:** This will minimize the infant's dose and is useful for long-acting drugs that can be given once daily.

9. **Temporarily Withhold Breastfeeding:** Depending on the estimated length of drug therapy, nursing can be temporarily withheld. Mothers may

be able to pump a sufficient quantity of milk beforehand for use during therapy. The pharmacokinetics of the drug must be examined to determine when the resumption of breastfeeding is advisable.

10. **Discontinue Nursing**: A few drugs are too toxic to allow nursing and may be necessary for the mother's health.

References

Chapter 1: An Overview of Medications and Pregnancy: Current Concepts

(1) Statistic Brain Research Institute. *Pregnancy Statistics*. Retrieved from http://statisticbrain.com/pregnancy-statistics/.

(2) Centers for Disease Control and Prevention. *Drugs and Statistics. Treating for Two. Medications and Pregnancy*. Retrieved from http://www.cdc.gov/pregnancy/meds/treatingfortwo/data/html..

(3) Keegan, J., Parva, M., Finnegan, M., Gerson, A., & Belden M. (2010). Addiction in pregnancy. *Journal of Addictive Diseases, 29*(2), 175-191.

(4) Reece-Stremtan, S., & Marinelli, K.A. (2015). ABM Clinical Protocol #21: Guidelines for breastfeeding and substance use or substance use disorder, revised 2015. *Breastfeeding Medicine, 10*(3), 135-141.

(5) Vaiserman AM. (2015). Early-life exposure to substance abuse and risk of Type 2 Diabetes in adulthood. *Current Diabetes Reports, 15*(48), 1-7.

(6) Nice, F.J. (2015, Nov.). *PHAR 622 Pharmacotherapy and Medication Management Endocrinology and Urology Syllabus Course: Medication Use in Pregnancy and Lactation*. University of Maryland Eastern Shore School of Pharmacy.

Chapter 2: An Overview of Medications and Breastfeeding: Current Concepts

(1) Nice, F.J., & Luo, A.C. (2015). Medications and breastfeeding: current concepts. *Journal of the American Pharmacists Association, 52*(1), 86-94.

(2) Bonyata, K. *Exercise and Breastfeeding*. Retrieved from http://kellymom.com/bf/can-i-breastfeed/lifestyle/mom-exercise/.

(3) Jensen, A.A, & Slorach, S.A. (1991). *Chemical Contaminants in Human Milk*. Boca Raton: CRC Press.

(4) Cohen, M. (2007). Environmental toxins and health: the health impact of pesticides. *Australian Family Physician, 36*(12), 1002-1004.

(5) Rogan, W.J., Bagniewska, A., & Damstra, T. (1980). Pollutants in breast milk. *New England Journal of Medicine, 302*(26), 1450-1453.

(6) Vaiserman, A.M. (2015). Early-life exposure to substance abuse and risk of Type 2 Diabetes in adulthood. *Current Diabetes Reports, 15*(48), 1-7.

(7) Wishart, D.S., Knox, C., Guo, A.C., Cheng, D., Shrivastava, S., Tzur, D., Hassanali M. (2008). DrugBank: a knowledgebase for drugs, drug actions and drug targets. *Nucleic Acids Research, 36*(Database Issue), D901-906.

(8) National Center for Biotechnology Information. U.S. National Library of Medicine. *The PubChem Project*. Retrieved from Pubchem.ncbi.nlm.nih.gov.

(9) Anderson PO. *LactMed*. Retrieved from

http://toxnet.nlm.nih.gov/cgi-bin/sis/htmlgen?LACT.

(10) Becker B. Hartman Group. *One-Third of U.S. Consumers Buying Organic, According to New Hartman Group Study*. Retrieved from http://www.hartman-group.com/.

(11) U.S. Food and Drug Administration. *Pregnancy and Lactation Labeling Final Rule*. Retrieved from http://www.fda.gov/Drugs/DevelopmentApprovalProcess/Develo pmentResources/Labeling/ucm093307.htm.

(12) Frolich, S., Stebbins, T.C., & Sauter, M.B. *The Next 11 States to Legalize Marijuana*. Retrieved from http://www.usatoday.com/story/money/business/2015/08/18/24-7-wall-st-marijuana/31834875/.

(13) Drugs.com. *Commonly Abused Drugs and Substances: Marijuana*.

Retrieved from www.drugs.com/illicit/marijuana.html.

Chapter 3: A List of Controlled Substances

(1) National Institute on Drug Abuse (NIDA). *The Science of Drug Abuse & Addiction. Commonly Abused Drugs Charts*. Retrieved from http://drugabuse.gov/drugs-abuse/common.

(2) US Drug Enforcement Agency (DEA), Office of Diversion Control. *Controlled Substance Schedules and List of Controlled Substances*.

Retrieved from

http://www.deadiversion.isdoj.gov/schdule/.

(3) US Drug Enforcement Agency (DEA), Office of Diversion Control. *Controlled Substance Drug Scheduling*. Retrieved from http://www.dea.gov/druginfor/ds/shtml.

(4) U.S. National Library of Medicine. *TOXNET*. Retrieved from http://toxnet.nlm.nih.gov/.

(5) Drugs.com. *Commonly Abused Drugs and Substances: Marijuana*.

Retrieved from www.drugs.com/illicit/marijuana.html.

Chapter 4: A Review of ABM Protocol #21 and List of Breastfeeding Questions for Healthcare Professionals

(1) Jansson, L.M. (2009). ABM Clinical Protocol #21: Guidelines for breastfeeding and the drug-dependent woman. *Breastfeeding Medicine, 4*(4), 225-228.

(2) Reece-Stremtan, S., & Marinelli, K.A. (2015). ABM Clinical Protocol #21: Guidelines for breastfeeding and substance use or substance use disorder, revised 2015. *Breastfeeding Medicine, 10*(3), 135-141.

(3) Baby-Friendly USA. *Baby-Friendly Hospital Initiative*. Retrieved from https://www.babyfriendlyusa.org/about-us/baby-friendly-hospital-initiative.

Chapter 5: Schedule I Drugs

(1) US Drug Enforcement Agency (DEA), Office of Diversion Control. *Controlled Substance Schedules and List of Controlled Substances*.

Retrieved from http://www.deadiversion.isdoj.gov/schdule/.

(2) US Drug Enforcement Agency (DEA), Office of Diversion Control. *Controlled Substance Drug Scheduling*. Retrieved from http://www.dea.gov/druginfor/ds/shtml.

(3) Keegan, J., Parva, M., Finnegan, M., Gerson, A., & Belden M. (2010). Addiction in pregnancy. *Journal of Addictive Diseases, 29*(2), 175-191.

(4) National Institute on Drug Abuse. *The Science of Drug Abuse & Addiction. Commonly Abused Drugs Charts*. Retrieved from http://drugabuse.gov/drugs-abuse/common.

(5) Greinwald, J.H. Jr, & Hotel, M.R. (1996). Absorption of topical cocaine in rhinologic procedures. *Laryngoscope, 106*(10), 1223-1225.

Chapter 6: Marijuana

(1) Anderson, L. *CSA Schedules*. Retrieved from http:www.drugs.com/csa-schedule.html.

(2) Integrative Addiction Medicine Institute. *Regular Cannabis Use Causes Loss in Brain Volume*. Retrieved from http://integrativeaddictioninstitute.awaremed.com/cannabis-use.

(3) King's College London. *Pharmaceutical Processing. Brain damage caused by cannabis?* Retrieved from http://www.pharmpro.com/printpdf/news/2015/11/brain-damage-caused-cannabis.

(4) National Institute on Drug Abuse (NIDA). *The Science of Drug Abuse & Addiction. Commonly Abused Drugs Charts*. Retrieved from http://drugabuse.gov/drugs-abuse/common.

(5) Vega, C.P. *Marijuana use associated with substantial adverse events CME/CE*. Retrieved from www.medscape.org/viewarticle/829278.

(6) Volkow, N.D., Baler, R.D., Compton, W.M., & Weiss, S.R.B. (2014). Adverse health effects of marijuana use. *The New England Journal of Medicine, 370*, 2219-2227.

(7) Fried, P.A. (2002). The consequences of marijuana use during pregnancy: a review of the human literature. *Journal of Cannabis Therapeutics, 2*(3/4), 86.

(8) Jacques, S.C., Kingsbury, A., Henshcke, P., Chomchai, C., Clews, S., Falconer, J., Oei, J.L. (2014). Cannabis, the pregnant woman and weeding out the myths. *Journal of Perinatology, 34*(6), 417-424.

(9) Lester, B., Andreozzi, L., & Appiahm, L. (2004). Substance abuse during pregnancy: time for policy to catch up with research. *Harm Reduction Journal, 1*(5), 13.

(10) US Drug Enforcement Agency (DEA), Office of Diversion Control. *Controlled Substance Schedules and List of Controlled Substances*.

Retrieved from http://www.deadiversion.isdoj.gov/schdule/.

(11) US Drug Enforcement Agency (DEA), Office of Diversion Control. *Controlled Substance Drug Scheduling*. Retrieved from http://www.dea.gov/druginfor/ds/shtml.

(12) Geppert, C.M.A. (2014). Legal and Clinical evolution of Veterans Health Administration policy on medical marijuana. *Federal Practitioner, 31*(3), 7-12.

(13) Gogek, E. *Marijuana debunked: the case against legalization.* Retrieved from http://www.mercatornet.com/articles/view/marijuana-debunked-the-case-against-legalization/16827.

(14) Tanner, L. (2015). *Pharmaceutical Processing. Scant evidence that medical pot helps many illnesses.* Retrieved from http://www.pharmpro.com/news/2015/06/study-scant-evidence-medical-pot-helps-many-illnesses.

(15) Friedman, D., & Devinsky, O. (2015). Cannabinoids in the treatment of epilepsy. *The New England Journal of Medicine, 373,* 1048-1058.

(16) Rosenberg, E.C., Tsien, R.W., Whalley, B.J., & Devinsky, O. (2015). Cannabinoids and Epilepsy. *Journal of the American Society for Experimental Neurotherapeutics,* Online: DOI 10.1007/s13311-015-0375-5.

Chapter 7: Schedule II, III, IV, IV and Non-Schedule Drugs

(1) National Institute on Drug Abuse (NIDA). *The Science of Drug Abuse & Addiction. Commonly Abused Drugs Charts.* Retrieved from http://drugabuse.gov/drugs-abuse/common.

(2) Nice, F.J. (2015, Nov.) *Pharmacotherapy and Medication Management Endocrinology and Urology Syllabus Course: Medication Use in Pregnancy and Lactation,* University of Maryland Eastern Shore School of Pharmacy PHAR 622.

(3) US Drug Enforcement Agency (DEA), Office of Diversion Control. *Controlled Substance Schedules and List of Controlled Substances.*

Retrieved from http://www.deadiversion.isdoj.gov/schdule/.

(4) US Drug Enforcement Agency (DEA), Office of Diversion Control. *Controlled Substance Drug Scheduling.* Retrieved from http://www.dea.gov/druginfor/ds/shtml.

(5) Keegan, J., Parva, M., Finnegan, M., Gerson, A., & Belden, M. (2010). Addiction in pregnancy. *Journal of Addictive Diseases, 29*(2), 175-191.

(6) Hastrup, M.B., Pottegard, A., & Damkier, P. (2014). Alcohol and breastfeeding. *Basic & Clinical Pharmacology & Toxicology, 114*(2), 168-173.

(7) Polygenis, D., Wharton, S., Malmbert, C., Sherman, N., Kennedy, D., Koren, G., & Einarson, T.R. (1998). Moderate alcohol consumption during pregnancy and the incidence of fetal malformations: a meta-analysis. *Neurotoxicology and Teratology, 20*(1), 61.

(8) Substance Abuse and Mental Health Services Administration. *Results from the 2012 National Health Survey on Drug Use and Health: Summary of National Findings, NSDUH Series H-46, HHS Publication No. (SMA) 13-4795. Current alcohol use among pregnant women in the US, 2011-2012, 2013:33.* Rockville, MD: Substance Abuse and Mental Health Services Administration.

(9) Chomchai, C., Chomchai, S., & Kitsommart. R. Transfer of methamphetamine (MA) into breast milk and urine of postpartum women who smoked MA tablets during pregnancy: implications for initiation of breastfeeding. *Journal of Human Lactation.* Retrieved from http://intl.jhl.sagepub.com/content/early/2015/10/09/0890334415 610080.abstract.

(10) National Institute on Drug Abuse (NIDA). *The Science of Drug Abuse & Addiction. Drug Facts: Anabolic Steroids.* Retrieved from http://drugabuse.gov/publications/drugfacts/anabolic-steroids.

(11) Su, P.H., Chang, Y.Z., & Chen, J.Y. (2010). Infant with in utero ketamine exposure: quantitative measurement of residual dosage in hair. *Pediatric Neonatology, 51*(5), 279-284.

(12) Zuccarini, P. (2009). Camphor: risks and benefits of a widely used natural product. *Journal of Applied Sciences and Environmental Management, 13*(2):69-74.

(13) Center for Substance Abuse Research. *Dextromethorphan (DXM).* Retrieved from File://C:/Users/Owner/Desktop/Dextromethorphan%20(DXM)% 20_%20CESAR.html.

(14) Drugs.com. *Meprobamate.* Retrieved from http://www.drugs.com/pro/meprobamate.html.

(15) National Eating Disorders Association. *Bulimia Nervosa.* Retrieved from https://www.nationaleatingdisorders.org/bulimia-nervosa.

(16) Rose, G. *Health risks of HGH.* Retrieved from http://livestrong.com/article/212121-health-risks-of-high/ (Note sections on acromegaly, acquired Creutzfeldt-Jakob disease, and breast enlargement and tumors).

(17) Reeves, R.R., Burke, R.S., & Kose, S. (2012). Carisoprodol: update on abuse potential and legal status. *Southern Medical Journal, 105*(11), 619-623.

(18) Futures of Palm Beach. *Cyclobenzaprine Abuse and Treatment.* Retrieved from http://futuresofplmbeach.com/cyclobenzaprine-treatment/ (Note only information for skeletal muscle relaxants abuse and signs of addiction).

Chapter 8: Neonatal Abstinence Syndrome (NAS)

(1) Kandall, S. R. (1996). *Substance and Shadow: A History of Women and Addiction in the United States—1850 to the present.* Cambridge, MA: Harvard University Press.

(2) Marcellus, L. (2007). Neonatal abstinence syndrome: Reconstructing the evidence. Neonatal Network, 26(1), 33-40.

(3) Marshall, O. (1878).The opium habit in Michigan. *Michigan State Board of Health Annual Report, 6,* 63-73, Reproduced in O'Donnell, J. A., and Ball, J. C. (1966) *Narcotic Addiction.* New York: J. & J. Harper Editions, pp. 45-54.

(4) Pettey, G. E. (1913). *Narcotic Drug Diseases and Allied Ailments.* Tennessee: J. A. Davis.

(5) Behnke, M., & Smith, V.C. (2013). Committee on Substance Abuse and Committee on Fetus and Newborn. Prenatal substance abuse: short- and long-term effects on the exposed fetus. *Pediatrics, 131,* e1009-e, 1024.

(6) Hudak, M.L., & Tan, R.C. (2012). Committee on Drugs and Committee of Fetus and Newborn Clinical Report: Neonatal drug withdrawal. *Pediatrics, 129*(2), e540-e560.

(7) Jansson, L.M., Svikis, D., Lee, J., Paluzzi, P., Rutigliano, P., & Hackerman, F. (1996). Pregnancy and addiction: a comprehensive care model. *Journal of Substance Abuse Treatment, 13*(4), 321-329.

(8) Ordean, A., & Kahan, M. (2011). Comprehensive treatment program for pregnant substance users in a family medicine clinic. *Canadian Family Physician, 57,* e430-5.

(9) World Health Organization (2014). Guidelines for the identification and management of substance use and substance use disorders in pregnancy. Geneva (Switzerland): World Health Organization. Retrieved from http://www.who.int/substance_abuse/publications/pregnancy_guidelines/en/.

(10) American Congress of Obstetricians and Gynecologists (ACOG). ACOG's Clinical Guidelines accessed at http://www.acog.org/About-ACOG/ACOG-Departments/Deliveries-Before-39-Weeks/ACOG-Clinical-Guidelines.

(11) Reese-Stremtan, S., Marinelli, K.A., & The Academy of Breastfeeding Medicine (2015). ABM Clinical Protocol #21: Guidelines for breastfeeding and substance use or substance use disorder, revised 2015. *Breastfeeding Medicine, 10*(3), 135-141.

(12) Jones, H.E., Kaltenbach, K., Heil, S., Stine, S.M., Coyle, M.G., Arria, A.M., & Fischer, G. (2010). Neonatal abstinence syndrome after methadone or buprenorphine exposure. *The New England Journal of Medicine, 363*, 2320-2331.

(13) Pierog S., Chandavasu O., & Wexler, I. (1977). Withdrawal symptoms in infants with the fetal alcohol syndrome. *Journal of Pediatrics, 90*, 630–633.

(14) Robe, L. B., Gromisch, D. S., & Iosub, S. (1980). Symptoms of neonatal ethanol withdrawal. *Currents in alcoholism, 8*, 485-493.

(15) Law, K.L., Stroud, L.R., LaGasse, L.L., Niaura, R., Liu. J., & Lester, B.M. (2003). Smoking during pregnancy and newborn neurobehavior. *Pediatrics, 111*(6), 1318-1323.

(16) Beauman, S.S. (2005). Identification and management of neonatal abstinence syndrome. *Journal of Infusion Nursing, 28*(3), 159-167.

(17) Jansson, L.M. & Velez, M. (2011). Infants of drug-dependent mothers. *Pediatrics in Review, 32*(1), 5-13.

(18) Klinger, G., & Merlob, P. (2008). Selective serotonin reuptake inhibitor induced neonatal abstinence syndrome. *The Israel journal of psychiatry and related sciences, 45*(2), 107-113.

(19) Calvigioni, D., Hurd, Y.L., Harkany, T., & Kiempema, E. (2014). Neuronal substrates and functional consequences of prenatal cannabis exposure. European Child & Adolescent Psychiatry, 23, 931-941.

(20) Velez, M., & Jansson, L.M. (2008). The opioid dependent mother and newborn dyad: nonpharmacologic care. *Journal of Addiction Medicine, 2*(3), 113-120.

(21) Fischer, G., Johnson, R.E., Eder, H., Jagsch, R., Peternell, A., Weninger, M., & Aschauer H.N. (2000). Research Report: Treatment of opioid-dependent pregnant women with buprenorphine. *Addiction, 95*(2), 239-244.

(22) Welle-Strand, G.K., Skurtveit, S., Jones, H.E., Waal, H., Bakstad, B., Bjarko, L., & Ravndal, E. (2013). Neonatal outcomes following in utero exposure to methadone or buprenorphine: A national cohort study of opioid-agonist treatment of pregnant women in Norway from 1996 to 2009. *Drug and Alcohol Dependence, 127*, 200-206.

(23) National Library of Medicine's TOXNET System. *LactMed: A New NLM Database on Drugs and Lactation.* Retrieved from http://toxnet.nlm.nih.gov/newtoxnet/lactmed.htm

(24) Pritham, U.A. (2013). Breastfeeding promotion for management of neonatal abstinence syndrome. *Journal of Obstetric, Gynecologic, and Neonatal Nursing, 42*, 517-526.

(25) Cleary, B.J., Donnelly, J., Strawbridge, J., Gallagher, P.J., Fahey, T., Clarke, M., & Murphy, D.J. (2010). Methadone dose and neonatal abstinence syndrome - systematic review and meta-analysis. *Addiction, 105*, 2071-2084.

(26) U.S. Food and Drug Administration (FDA, 2013). Information for Healthcare Professionals: Methadone Hydrochloride text version. Retrieved from: http://www.fda.gov/Drugs/DrugSafety/PostmarketDrugSafetyInformationforPatientsandProviders/ucm142841.htm

(27) Jansson, L.M., Choo, R.E., Harrow, C., Velez, M., Schroeder, J.R., Lowe, R., & Huestis, M.A. (2007). Concentrations of methadone in breast milk and plasma in the immediate perinatal period. *Journal of Human Lactation, 23*(2), 184-190.

(28) Jansson, L.M., DiPietro, J.A., Elko, A., Williams, E.L., Milio, L., & Velez, M. (2012). Pregnancies exposed to methadone, methadone and other illicit substances, poly-drugs without methadone: A comparison of fetal neurobehaviors and infant outcomes. *Drug and Alcohol Dependence, 122*, 213-219.

(29) Popova, S., Lange, S., Shield, K., Mihic, A., Chudley, A.E., Mukherjee, R.S., Kekmuradov, D., & Rehm, J. (2016). Comorbidity of fetal alcohol spectrum disorder: A systematic review and meta-analysis. *Lancet, 387*, 978-87.

(30) Mennella, J.A., & Beauchamp, G.K. (1991). The transfer of alcohol to human milk – Effects on flavor and the infant's behavior. *The New England Journal of Medicine, 325*(14), 981-85.

(31) Narkowicz, S., Plotka, J., Polkowski, Z., Biziuk, & Namiesnik, J. (2013). Prenatal exposure to substance of abuse: A worldwide problem. Environment International, 54, 141-163.

(32) Smith, L., Yonekura, M.L., Wallace, T., Berman, N., Kuo, J., & Berkowitz, C. (2003). Effects of prenatal methamphetamine exposure on fetal growth and drug withdrawal symptoms in infants born at term. *Developmental and Behavioral Pediatrics, 24*(1), 17-23.

(33) Kiblaw, Z.N., Smith, L.M., Diaz, S.D., LaGasse, L., Derauf, C., Newman, E., & Lester, B. (2014). Prenatal methamphetamine exposure and neonatal and infant neurobehavioral outcome: Results from the IDEAL study. *Substance Abuse, 35*, 68-73.

(34) Oei, J.L., Kingsbury, A., Dhawan, A., Burns, L., Feller, J.M., Clews, S., Falconer, J., & Abdel-Latif, M.E. (2012). Amphetamines, the pregnant woman and her children: a review. *Journal of Perinatology, 32*, 737-747.

(35) Bartu, A., Dusci, L.J., & Ilett, K.F. (2008). Transfer of methylamphetamine and amphetamine into breast milk following recreational use of methylamphetamine. *British Journal of Clinical Pharmacology, 67*(4), 455-459.

(36) Iqbal, M.M., Sobhan, T., & Ryals (2002). Effects of commonly used benzodiazepines on the fetus, the neonate, and the nursing infant. *Psychiatric Services,53*(1), 39-49.

(37) Kelly, L.E., Poon, S., Madadi, P., & Koren, G. (2012). Neonatal benzodiazepines exposure during breastfeeding. *The Journal of Pediatrics,161*, 448-51.

(38) Rubin, E.T., Lee, A., & Ito, S. (2004). When breastfeeding mothers need CNS-acting drugs. *Canadian Journal of Clinical Pharmacology, 11*(2), e257-266.

(39) Castellanos, F.X., & Rapoport, J.L. (2002). Effects of caffeine on development and behavior in infancy and childhood: a review of the published literature. Food and Chemical Toxicology, 40, 1235-1242.

(40) So, M., Bozzo, P., Inoue, M., & Einarson, A. (2010). Safety of antihistamines during pregnancy and lactation. *Canadian Family Physician, 56*(5), 427-429.

(41) Mansi, G., Raimondi, F., Pichini, S., Capasso, L., Sarnp, M., & Paludetto, R. (2007). Neonatal urinary cotinine correlates with behavioral alterations in newborns prenatally exposed to tobacco smoke. *Pediatric Research, 61*(2), 257–261.

(42) Mennella, J.A., Yourshaw, L.M., & Morgan, L.K. (2007). Breastfeeding and smoking: Short-term effects on infant feeding and sleep. *Pediatrics, 120*(3), 497-512.

(43) Menon, S.J. (2008). Psychotropic medication during pregnancy and lactation. *Archives of Gynecology and Obstetric, 277*, 1-13.

(44) Fortinguerra, F., Clavenna, A., & Bonati, M. (2009). Psychotropic drug use during breastfeeding: A review of the evidence. *Pediatrics, 124*(4), e547-e556.

(45) Lanza di Scalea, T., & Wisnes, K. (2009). Antidepressant medication use during breastfeeding. *Clinical Obstetrics and Gynecology, 52*(3), 483-497.

(46) Lange, S., Shield, K., Koren, G., Rehm, J., & Popova, S. (2014). A comparison of the prevalence of prenatal alcohol exposure obtained via maternal self-reports versus meconium testing: A systematic literature review and meta-analysis. *BMC Pregnancy & Childbirth, 14*:127.

(47) United States Drug Testing Laboratories (USDTL), INC. *The perinatal testing group*. Retrieved from

http://www.usdtl.com/perinatal-testing/testing-group.

(48) Pritham, U.S. (2013). Management of neonatal abstinence syndrome. *Journal of Obstetric, Gynecologic, and Neonatal Nursing, 42*, 517-26.

(49) Jansson, L.M., Spencer, N., McConnell, K., Velez, M., Harrow, C.A, Jones, H.E., Swortwood, M.J., Barnes, B.S., Scheidweiler, K.B., & Huestis, M.A. (in press). Maternal Buprenorphine Maintenance and Lactation. *Journal of Human Lactation*, in press.

(50) Lindemalm, S., Nydert, P., Svensson, J., Stahle, L., & Sarman, I. (2009). Transfer of buprenorphine into breastmilk and calculation of infant drug dose. *Journal of Human Lactation, 25*(2), 199-205.

(51) Finnegan, L., Connaughton, J., Kron, R., Emich, J. (1975). Neonatal abstinence syndrome: assessment and management. *Journal of Addictive Diseases, 2*, 141-158.

(52) Velez, M., & Jansson, L.M. (2008). The opioid dependent mother and newborn dyad: non-pharmacologic care. *Journal of Addiction Medicine, 2*(3), 113-120.

(53) Abbett, H., & Greenwood, S. (2012). Nursing infants with neonatal abstinence syndrome: Time to change practice? *Journal of Neonatal Nursing, 18*(6), 194-197.

(54) Jansson, L.M., Velez, M., & Harrow, C. (2009). The opioid-exposed newborn: Assessment and pharmacologic management. *Journal of Opioid Management, 5*(1), 7-55.

(55) Baldacchino, A., Arbuckle, K., Petrie, D.J., & McCowan, C. (2014). Neurobehavioral consequences of chronic intrauterine opioid exposure in infants and pre-school children: a systematic review and meta-analysis. *BMC Psychiatry, 14:104.*

(56) March of Dimes (2003). Understanding the behavioral of term newborns: States of the term newborn. *Perinatal Nursing Education.* Retrieved from: www.marchofdimes.org/nursing/modnemedia/othermedia/states.pdf

(57) Colson, S. (2012). Biological nurturing: The laid-back breastfeeding revolution. Retrieved from: http://www.biologicalnurturing.com/assets/MT101BioNurtpdf.pdf

(58) Genna, C.W., & Barak, D. (2010). Facilitating autonomous infant hand use during breastfeeding. *Clinical Lactation, 1, 13-18.*

Chapter 9: Treatment Drugs

(1) National Institute on Drug Abuse (NIDA). *Principles of Drug Treatment: A Research-Based Guide (Third Edition): Evidence-Based Approaches to Drug Addiction.* Retrieved from http://www.drugabuse.gov/publications/principles-drug-addiction-treatment-research-based-guide-third-edition/acknowledgments.

(2) Briggs, G.G., & Freeman, R.K. (2015). Drugs in Pregnancy and Lactation: A Reference Guide to Fetal and Neonatal Risk. Philadelphia: Wolters Kluver.

(3) Truven Health Analytics. (2012-2016). *Disulfiram*. Retrieved from www.micromedexsolutions.com.

(4) Truven Health Analytics. (2012-2016). *Methadone*. Retrieved from www.micromedexsolutions.com.

(5) Legal Information Institute. (2003). 42 CFR 8.12 - *Federal opioid treatment standards*. Retrieved from https://www.law.cornell.edu/cfr/text/42/8.12.

(6) Truven Health Analytics. (2012-2016). *Buprenorphine/Naloxone*. Retrieved from www.micromedexsolutions.com.

(7) Truven Health Analytics. (2012-2016). *Naloxone*. Retrieved from www.micromedexsolutions.com.

(8) Truven Health Analytics. (2012-2016). *Naltrexone*. Retrieved from www.micromedexsolutions.com.

Chapter 10: Counseling

(1) Indian Health Service (IHS). (n.d.). Tool 9. Pharmacist Consultation. *Health Literacy Toolkit*. Retrieved from http://www.ihs.gov/healthcommunications/documents/toolkit/Tool9.pdf.

(2) Indian Health Service (IHS). (n.d). *Patient Provider Toolkit*. Retrieved from http://www.ihs.gov/healthcommunications/index.cfm?module=dsp_hc_toolkit.

(3) Plain Language.gov. (n.d.) *Avoid Legal, Foreign, and Technical Jargon*. Retrieved from http://www.plainlanguage.gov/howto/guidelines/FederalPLGuidelines/writeNoJargon.cfm

(4) Levy, A.H. (2011). *The Falling Man: An Interview With Henry Singer*. Retrieved from http://designobserver.com/feature/the-falling-man-an-interview-with-henry-singer/30048/.

(5) Chen, A.M.H., Noureldin, M., & Plake, K.S. (2013). Impact of a health literacy assignment on student pharmacist learning. *Research in Social and Administrative Pharmacy, 9*(5), 531-541.

(6) Indian Health Service (IHS). (n.d.) Tool 19. Patient Goals. *Health Literacy Toolkit.* Retrieved from http://www.ihs.gov/healthcommunications/documents/toolkit/To o1l9.pdf.

(7) Berger, B.A., & Villaume, W.A. (2013). *What Is Motivational Interviewing? A Sensible Approach. Motivational Interviewing For Health Care Professionals: A Sensible Approach* (pp. 27-34). Washington DC: American Pharmacists Association.

(8) Center for Substance Abuse Treatment. (1999). Motivational Interviewing as a Counseling Style. In *Enhancing Motivation for Change in Substance Abuse Treatment. Treatment Improvement Protocol (TIP) Series, No. 35.* Rockville (MD): Substance Abuse and Mental Health Services Administration (US).

(9) Nice, F.J. Nice Flyers. *Counseling Tips.* Retrieved from http://www.nicebreastfeeding.com.

(10) Rx-wiki. (n.d.) Omnibus Budget Reconciliation Act of 1990. http://rx-wiki.org/index.php?title=Omnibus_Budget_Reconcilliation_Act.

(11) Streetdrugs.org. (2015). *Streetdrugs 2015*, 15th Ed. Long Lake MN: Publisher's Group West.

(12) Substance Abuse and Mental Health Services Administration. (2012). *Clinical Drug Testing in Primary Care.* Technical Assistance Publication (TAP) 32. Rockville, MD: Substance Abuse and Mental Health Services Administration.

(13) Lyttle, T. (2006). Stop the injustice: a protest against the unconstitutional punishment of pregnant drug-addicted women. *The New York University Journal of Legislation and Public Policy, 8*(2), 812-813.

Appendix 1: Controlled Drug Substances Schedules

(1) U.S. Drug Enforcement Agency (DEA). Office of Diversion Control. (n.d.). Controlled Substance Schedules and List of Controlled Substances. Retrieved from http://www.deadiversion.usdoj.gov/schedules/.

Appendix 2: Marijuana

(1) Anderson, L. (n.d.) *Marijuana*. Retrieved from www.drugs.com/illicit/marijuana.html.

(2) Anderson, L. (n.d.). *CSA Schedules*. Retrieved from http:www.drugs.com/csa-schedule.html.

(3) U.S. Drug Enforcement Agency (DEA). Office of Diversion Control. (n.d.). *Controlled Substance Schedules and List of Controlled Substances*. Retrieved from http://www.deadiversion.usdoj.gov/schedules/.

(4) Colorado Department of Public Health & Environment, Retail Marijuana Public Health Advisory Committee. (2014). *Monitoring the Health Concerns Related to Marijuana in Colorado: 2014*. Retrieved from https://www.colorado.gov/pacific/cdphe/retail-marijuana-public-health-advisory-committee.

(5) Washington State Government. *Initiative Measure No. 502*. Retrieved from sos.wa.gov/_assets/elections/initiatives/i502.pdf.

(6) Industry/Cannabis Industry Information for Businesses Including Tips, News, and Advice for Dispensaries. *Big Changes to Washington State's Medical Marijuana Program That Dispensaries Need to Know*. Retrieved from https://leafly.com/news/industry/new-licensing-requirements-for-....

Appendix 3: Recreational Drugs Use Recommendations for Breastfeeding

(1) Nice, F.J. Nice Flyers. *Counseling Tips*. Retrieved from http://www.nicebreastfeeding.com.

Appendix 4: Benefits of Breastfeeding and Risks of Not Breastfeeding

(1) Nice, F.J. Nice Flyers. *Counseling Tips*. Retrieved from http://www.nicebreastfeeding.com.

Appendix 5: Questions to Ask in Breastfeeding / Medication Situations

(1) Nice, F.J. Nice Flyers. *Counseling Tips*. Retrieved from http://www.nicebreastfeeding.com.

Appendix 6: Stepwise Approach to Minimize Infant Drug Exposure While Breastfeeding

(1) Nice, F.J. Nice Flyers. *Counseling Tips*. Retrieved from http://www.nicebreastfeeding.com.

Index

175

About the Authors

Frank J. Nice, RPh, DPA, CPHP

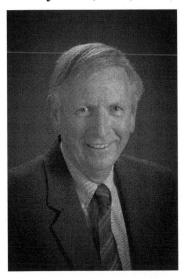

Dr. Frank J. Nice has practiced as a consultant, lecturer, and author on medications and breastfeeding for 40 years. He holds a Bachelor's Degree in Pharmacy, a Masters Degree in Pharmacy Administration, Master's and Doctorate Degrees in Public Administration, and Certification in Public Health Pharmacy. He retired from the US Public Health Service after 30 years of distinguished service. Dr. Nice practiced at the National Institutes of Health (NIH) and served as a Project Manager at the Food and Drug Administration (FDA). He recently retired after 43 years of government service and currently is self-employed as a consultant and President, Nice Breastfeeding LLC (www.nicebreastfeeding.com).

Dr. Nice has published *Nonprescription Drugs for the Breastfeeding Mother*, 2nd Edition and *The Galactogogue Recipe Book*. Dr. Nice has also authored over four dozen peer-reviewed articles on the use of prescription medications, Over-the-Counter (OTC) products, and herbals during breastfeeding, in addition to articles and book chapters on the use of power, epilepsy, and work characteristics of healthcare professionals. He has organized and participated in over 50 medical missions to the country of Haiti. Dr. Nice continues to provide consultations, lectures, and presentations to the breastfeeding community and to serve the poor of Haiti.

LCDR Amy C. Luo, RPh, PharmD

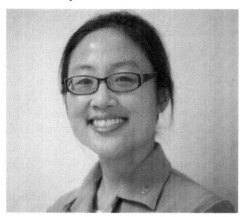

LCDR Amy C. Luo, USPHS is a pharmacist who works on the Navajo Reservation in Crownpoint, New Mexico. She holds a Doctorate of Pharmacy Degree from Rutgers University. Amy met Dr. Nice through her "Intermediate Pharmacy Practice Experience" (IPPE) at the National Institutes of Health (NIH). She then coauthored the article titled "Medications and Breastfeeding: Current Concepts." Amy plans to increase her experience caring for breastfeeding mothers during her professional career.

LCDR Luo has been serving as a pharmacist on the Reservation for five years. She worked in Kayenta, Arizona, before moving to Crownpoint. She calls Kayenta her "home on the rez." Kayenta is where she fell in love with the red rocks, the Diné (Navajo people), and being an Indian Health Service (IHS) pharmacist. She enjoys teaching, mentoring, and going on adventures with pharmacy students. Amy continues to serve the Diné as a pharmacist and mentors students as a preceptor.

Cheryl A. Harrow, DNP, FNP-BC, IBCLC

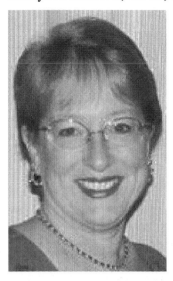

Dr. Cheryl A. Harrow enjoys teaching in the clinical setting and in the PhD, DNP, and MSN programs at Catholic University (CUA). Before joining the CUA School of Nursing, she was clinical faculty for the undergraduate and accelerated programs at Johns Hopkins University School of Nursing. She continues to precept nurse practitioner students in the Newborn Nursery at Johns Hopkins Bayview Medical Center as adjunct faculty for the Johns Hopkins University School of Nursing, University of Maryland School of Nursing, Frontier Nursing University, and Walden University. Dr. Harrow demonstrates her devotion to teaching in her workplace using an interprofessional education model to share knowledge with registered nurses, nursing and medical students, and in collaboration with a team of nurse practitioners, physician assistants, pediatricians, and neonatologists.

Dear Reader,

Thank you for purchasing and reading this book. We hope you enjoyed it. If so, you can help us reach other readers by writing a review of the book on Amazon.com and / or www.nicebreastfeeding.com.

Sincerely,

Frank J. Nice & Amy C. Luo & Cheryl A. Harrow